# Native American Herbalism

*Everything you need to know about the Secret*

*Ancient Herbal Remedies from the fields*

*to your Apothecary table*

**MIGUELA SANCHEZ**

# Table of Contents

# CHAPTER FIVE: HERBAL REMEDIES & RECIPES.... 44

# INTRODUCTION

Before modern medicine, we relied heavily on "unrefined" herbal medicine to treat the different illnesses we came down with. The herbs weren't even put to any pharmaceutical modification before we, at that time, took them for one ailment or another. We either cooked or ground the herbs to break the plant components down making them edible before consuming them, and they always worked.

Fast forward to today, herbal medicine remains one of the only few highly effective medicinal remedies to the medical conditions we develop. Pharmaceutical companies still even use them in modern medicines for their scent, flavor and healing properties. If you even walk into any pharmacy today and buy a drug, there is a high chance you'll find these herbs in the tablets, capsules, powders, tea, extracts, etc. You purchase over the counter. These herbs are used in drug production because they contain strong substances that stimulate vigorous physiological and, certainly, medicinal activities in our body when we consume them.

The herbs found in Native America, particularly, have been confirmed to possess highly therapeutic substances and these have been further categorized, by experts, into the following: Alkaloids, Anthocyanins, Anthraquinones, Cardiac Glycosides, Coumarins, Cyanogenic Glycosides, Flavonoids, Glucosilinates, Phenols, Saponins, Tannins, etc.

All of these substances have the power to repair our tissues and organs and also provide your body with a long-lasting protection against recurring diseases and ailments.

Native American Medicine had been a major influence on modern medicine, even long before the Europeans came into the territory. It served the natives as remedies to many of the illnesses and conditions they experienced. These herbs still serve us today, and will continue to do so. It is for this reason that I have decided to dedicate a body of extensive research—and a period of thorough inquiry into the therapeutic properties of these herbs—to provide you with the necessary information about Native American herbs and their immense benefits when you use them as medicine to the conditions you may experience.

I'd like you to see this book as a definitive guide to all the Native American herbs you can ever find, anywhere. The fact you're holding this book at the moment suggests you already understand how powerful Native American medicine is and would like to explore the healing powers they provide. Well, you've done the right thing by acquiring this book and I'd like to congratulate you.

*Native American Herbalism* is the master key you need to unlock the deep secrets about the tremendous power Northern American herbs possess. I implore you to make continued use of it. Trust me; at the end of this book, you'll be so glad you devoured its contents. Not only is it informational, but quite an interesting read as well.

So, I wish you a happy reading.

# CHAPTER ONE: MODERN NATIVE AMERICAN MEDICINE

## Background

Native Americans are known all over the world for their herbal medicinal knowledge. Rumor has it that, in any 400 modern drugs you come across, there's a high probability that about 200 of them derived from Native American herbs. Many of the medicines we even take today have active ingredients that were extracted from Native American herbs like ampalaya, ginger, echinacea, etc. Not only are they used in drugs, you'll also find them in beauty products, hair creams and so on.

According to oral history, herbalism in Native America started well over 10,000 years ago. But, unfortunately, there's no credible historical documentation of the native American tribes activities until they came in contact with the Europeans in the 16th century. Now, all we have before this period is the orally transferred systems and beliefs that have been passed on, from generations to generations.

But, among the popular oral stories the natives tell, there's one story that particularly catches my attention. This is a story about how the natives discovered the healing powers of herbs. It is usually said that the natives adopted herbalism into their culture after observing animals. The story says they discovered the magical effects of roots and herbs when the animals they observed swiftly regained their health after consuming some herbs.

You may find this story implausible, but there's an element of truth in it. If you know much about American natives, then you'll know how big they are on "reasoning by verification." This is what Western philosophers refer to as empiricism (i.e., knowledge can only be acquired though experience). Their life of apparent dependency on plains, forests and coastal regions is another explanation we can give to back up this story.

Some Native Americans hate to share their traditional herbal knowledge to non-native Americans because of the way some people have lightly dismissed their herbalism and beliefs. Despite this, a larger percentage of them have been most generous to share their knowledge with other enthusiastic settlers and tourists and this has been a major reason for the worldwide popularity of Native American Medicine today.

## Medicinal Properties in Native American Herbs

It is important we go through the healing agents you can find in these herbs together to give you a full understanding of how these herbs work and how you can best use them as remedies to certain illnesses.

It is the natural components in plants that are responsible for the healing effects we experience. These components are now recognized, in modern medicine, as minerals, vitamins, phytochemicals and enzymes. I've been going on and on about the medicinal properties of native American herbs since the beginning of this book—how they are the power of these herbs—and now you must be wondering, "what are these herbal medicinal properties?" Under this section, we'll examine all of them one after the other. So, get ready to learn the properties of American native herbs that bring about the therapeutic effects we experience.

# Phytochemicals

Phytochemicals can as well be referred to as plant chemicals since "phyto" means plants. These chemicals function as antioxidants, immune system strengtheners, enzyme secretion stimulants, plaque destroyers in blood vessels, and so much more when consumed.

Below are some of the plant chemicals that are highly concentrated in native American herbs:

- **Alkaloids**

This is one of the largest groups of medicinal properties. You'll always find it in one plant or another. They're virtually in every food, drink and supplements we take today. Neuroactive molecules like nicotine and caffeine, which are commonly consumed by all today, fall under this group. Emetine, vinblastine and vincristine are other alkaloid types you'll find in many native American plants as well. Two out of the long list of plants that are high in alkaloids are goldenseal and nightshades and these work in ousting toxicity from the body and fortifying our body's defense system.

- **Anthocyanins**

Anthocyanins are natural pigments that cause alternative colors in plants, vegetables, fruits and grains. Any herb you find in blue, red, a red-purple color, purple, and violet, is high in anthocyanins. Echinacea, which has been described as the most popular and widely used native American herbs in the US, contain high constituents of anthocyanins.

Anthocyanins build up the body's defense against free radicals, a substance that's produced after metabolic reactions have been triggered. This material can result in serious conditions like cancer or cardiovascular disease.

Anthocyanins also hinder the development of plaque in the bloodstream, stabilize blood flow and reduce the risk of developing cardiovascular disease. They can also be great at improving your vision, fighting edema and inflammation.

- **Chlorophyll**

We all know the function of chlorophyll in plants but not many of us know the benefit of this plant asset to us as humans. Chlorophyll is what is responsible for the greenness in plants. It ensures the absorption of sunlight and is a vital part of photosynthesis.

In humans, chlorophyll performs a completely different role. It:
- helps fights bacteria;
- helps to nicely heal wounds and burns
- helps to fight cancer.
- is a great source of vitamin K as well. Vitamin K helps to improve the skin and also strengthen your bones.

- **Diterpenes**

Diterpenes can also be found in most herbal plants. Among them are Bertoni and Rosemary that are potent detoxifiers, anti-inflammatory agents, anticancer agents, abnormal growth inducers, and antioxidants when consumed.

- **Eleutherosides**

Need to refresh yourself or boost your energy and overall health? Then, a good source of energy would be from any plant that has a high concentration of eleutherosides. Follow the preparation instructions and take as prescribed. Your stamina, even your mental alertness will be boosted immediately.

Eleutherosides also increases your appetite, improves your immune system as well as your mental system, and stimulates body metabolism. It's commonly used to cure menopause problems like hot flashes, irregular periods, etc.

- **Fatty Acids (Essential)**

There are only 2 essential fatty acids. And these are: omega-3 (alpha-linolenic acid) and omega-6 (linoleic acid) fatty acid. Other types are regarded as "conditionally essential" because they become "essential" only when we experience some diseases or some developments.

These essential fatty acids are important for good health but the body cannot break them down. So, all we have is these herbs that we must ingest to gain access to these valuable acids.

Below are the few functions they perform in the body:

- They make sure the cell membranes and of myelin sheaths (nerve fibers coverings) are in shape at all times.
- They stimulate the secretion of hormonelike substances called prostaglandin. These substances increase your immunity and also speed up body metabolism. In addition, they also help to ensure smooth nerve transmission &

muscle activity while at the same time maintaining low blood cholesterol levels.

You'll find them in several herbs but one of which is the popular palmetto plant.

- **Flavonglycosides**

This plant chemical is a potent antioxidant. It works in removing plaques in the blood vessel, improving blood flow; improving sight and hearing and enhancing mental ability. Flavonglycosides is also a powerful antidepressant. Ginkgo biloba is one plant where you can get this substance.

- **Gingerols**

Gingerols is an active substance in ginger (you might have guessed from the name). This is the herbal substance responsible for digestive system improvement. When you consume any gingerols-heavy plant, your digestive tracts will find it quite easy to break down fats, proteins and also transfer nutrients to every part in the body. This antioxidant fights liver toxicity as well.

- **Ginkolic Acid**

This is another potent antioxidant found in several Native American herbs. Imagine a multiple-in-one package. Yes, that's exactly what this plant chemical is: it provides improved blood circulation, sharpens mental clarity, lowers the risk of developing degenerative diseases, and fights cancer.

It also helps to relieve depression. So, on days you wake up on the wrong side of the bed, prepare and take a ginkgo biloba-heavy recipe and you'll feel a lot better.

- **Glycyrrhizins**

This is a chemical compound that's usually extracted from licorice and used in skin-care products for its anti-inflammatory, antiviral and skin repair properties.

- **Hesperidin**

Hesperidin works in strengthening body cell membranes and protecting your capillaries from damages. It's also used in fighting liver diseases like cirrhosis and hepatitis. Hesperidin also provides protection against damaging light rays and it can be gotten from milk thistle seeds.

- **Hypericin**

Hypericin is an antibiotic/antivirus/anti-depressant derivative of St. John's wort. This substance regulates the neurotransmitters in our mental system and has been used over the years in treating anxiety, depression and sleeping disorders.

- **Isothiocyanates**

This is another plant chemical commonly extracted from most Native American herbs. Isothiocyanates, which can be derived from horseradish, helps to stimulate protective enzymes secretion, prevent your DNA from damaging, and, in all, prevent & reduce the risk of cancer in any part of the body. They're particularly known for their anticarcinogenic tendency. Isothiocyanates hinder carcinogenesis and also facilitate detoxification. They have also been found to to fight tumors in a recent study carried out on this compound.

- **Lactones**

Lactones, like Isothiocyanates, are also anticarcinogenic. They reduce the risk of cancer in the body. They have also been confirmed to be skin sensitizers and can be gotten from the kava kava root.

## • Lipoic Acid

Lipoic acid is a strong antioxidant that is found in most herbs. This substance hinders the growth of and eliminates metals in the body. It helps in reducing skin roughness, reducing the risk of cancer, keeping blood sugar levels in check. They're also effective in treating inflammation, tiredness, heart diseases and even memory loss.

## • Phenolic Acids

Phenolic acids can be found in fruits, seeds, and fruit skins but are highly concentrated in plants, especially those native to the Americas. This acid is rich in antioxidants that inhibit oxidative stress, prevent cancer. It's also used in treating diabetes and heart diseases as well. You'll get them in parsley, berries and even in most plants you can find.

## • Phthalides

Phthalides are great detoxifiers of carcinogens. You'll find them in many drugs because they relax blood vessels to reduce blood pressure as well as increase blood flow. Phthalides also ensure essential enzymes needed for good health are produced.

## • Polyacetylenes

Polyacetylenes regulate the production of carcinogens and prostaglandins in the body.

## • Proanthocyanidins

Proanthocyanins provide protection against cancer, increase the strength of your blood vessel walls and balance your blood cholesterol. They're also a potent antioxidant for treating the influenza virus. You'll get them in bilberry, elderberry, etc.

- **Quercetin**

Quercetin is one of the flavonoids you'll find in several fruits, vegetables and herbs. Flavonoids are a type of antioxidants that naturally occur in plants. They're known for the anti-inflammation, anti-cancer properties and they also work well in protecting blood vessels and cell membranes from damage.

- **Rosmarinic Acid**

By now, you must have heard of this acid type before because they are highly popular and are usually the active ingredients in many modern drugs we consume.

They were extracted from rosemary plants and used in drug production because they work potently in improving digestive systems and fighting nausea. This phytochemical can also be quite effective in treating headaches and some other mild pains as well.

- **Salin**

When Hippocrates prescribed white willow barks and leaves to people, then he truly must have understood herbal medicine. A phytochemical called salicin (a.k.a salin) is contained in this plant. This compound, once ingested, helps to fight fever, pain and inflammation. It's highly effective for treating the influenza virus also.

- **Saponins**

Saponins have been used to make cough syrups, emetics, sneezing powders, etc., because they help to expel phlegm from your lungs. Why this is possible is because they're immediately inactivated by our cholesterin and this makes them only effective on our mucus membrane. They're also great anti-cancer agents.

- **Silymarin**

This another phytochemical derived from milk thistle. It's a potent antioxidant and it also ensures the optimal performance of our liver.

- **Tannins**

Tannins are common in virtually all plants. They are antioxidants and antiviral agents that improve the performance of your capillaries, reduce the risk of cancer, asthma and cardiovascular disease in your body system.

- **Terpenes**

Terpenes is the chemical responsible for the smell in cannabis plants. You can get them from Ginkgo biloba and ingesting them can also be great for your health. When occasionally consumed, they work as antioxidants. They also offer therapeutic effects similar to those you'd get from cannabinoids (THC & CBD).

- **Triterpenoids**

To treat ulcers, fight cancer and manage liver toxicity, you can consume recipes made from gotu kola and licorice roots. These plants are highly rich in triterpenoids and you can also use them to treat tooth decay as well.

## Enzymes

Enzymes are the "catalysts" of phytochemicals. For the phytochemicals, minerals and vitamins to function well in the body, they must be present. They are also necessary for the smooth absorption of the other properties contained in the herbs, which is why, like other herbal substances, they're ever present in plants. If you must live in good health, you'll need these enzymes in their original form. This is why you must ensure that any remedy you prepare mustn't be exposed to intense heat or alcohol, if you really want the best results.

## Benefits and Uses

We already highlighted the many benefits of using native American herbs in the previous section, but I feel it is necessary we go through them extensively so you can understand what you stand to gain from consuming these herbs instead of modern medicines.

Today, herbalism has improved so much that modern extraction methods have been adopted to speed up infusion and ensure the full harnessing of all the medicinal properties contained in the herbs. Even today, the principle idea behind most of the modern medicine we consume is taken from herbal medicine to then produce the drugs we purchase over the counter.

Native American herbs are used for a lot of things and their benefits are numerous. At the moment, we have not even exhausted the uses of the herbs that currently exist and there are millions of them yet to be discovered in native America and in other places as well. But, it'd be good to know some, if not all, of the benefits of using herbal medication.

Herbs are a great way to prevent cardiovascular diseases, cancer and other severe conditions that usually take regular and/or topical medicines to cure. They are naturally extracted and, in their fresh form, consumed. This then makes it easier for the herbal properties contained in the medicine to be properly absorbed into our systems so they can effectively serve their purpose and ultimately improve your health.

Herbs consumed without any modification are often more concentrated in antioxidants. So, when you consume them, your body will be able to quickly harness their therapeutic benefits and this results in a longer lifetime and a better health life.

Because modern medicines are often produced using different chemicals for preservation and what nots, they usually pose more adverse effects than herbal remedies. But, with herbs, the risk of exposure to side effects is considerably low. Not only do you get quicker results with the herbs, but also reduce negative effects when you consume them.

# Conclusion

It is certain native Americans didn't know what the medicinal properties of the plants they consumed were when they were using the herbs in those days. Today, many of them would still not know if you ask them. It's not because they didn't understand the herbs. They did. But, at that time, there was no simple way to know these things. What mattered to them at that time was that the herbs worked and they really enjoyed their benefits a great deal.

If you go through history, you'll find out that these native truly understood the herb type to use whenever they had an ailment and it has worked for them over the years. For example, whenever the natives came down with, say, a headache, they knew the plant they had to use, like Rosemary. What they didn't, however, know is medicinal properties—or healing agents—like the rosmarinic acid that causes the headache to subside.

# CHAPTER TWO: HOW TO SOURCE AND STORE HERBS

## Gathering Herbs The Right Way

As unbelievable as this can be, many people still don't know the right way to source quality herbs, and this is usually one of the many reasons for which the herbal remedies made and consumed don't work as they should. Most times, this leads the people using them incorrectly to completely give up on herbal remedies all together, particularly because they do not know where to find quality herbs or how to grow them. And this, to me, is just like giving up on great health—on the most minimal costs.

For people who are even new to herbal medication, herbs sourcing can be a lot of work. I'm sure, by now, you must already have been wondering, "what then is the right way to source herbs?" Frankly speaking, there's really no particularly special way to source quality herbs.

Contrary to the picture Harry Potter and some other fantasy novels might have painted for you, you really don't have to make life-threatening trips into the most mystical locations to collect powerful herbal plants. Herbs are not magical items needed to make potions. They're actually scientific—and have been proven to work effectively in treating many conditions.

You only need to understand a few crucial things such as, the right time to harvest, the exact plant parts to harvest and so many other details we'll discuss soon, to be able to effectively harness the therapeutic benefits these herbal medicines will give you.

## Buying

Due to their popularity, Native American herbs are sold virtually everywhere. You really don't have to make long, stressful trips to where the natives are, like Arizona, California, Oklahoma or Alaska, or other regions the tribes live, to get these herbs. Instead, you might want to search locally for the herbs in stores near you. If you can confirm they have high quality herbs in stock, then you shouldn't hold back from buying.

There are a few other factors you have to consider when you want to purchase native American herbs from a local producer or seller. These are:

- The quality of soil used in growing them;
- The method of cultivation;
- The way the herbs have been processed or dried;
- The method of storage used by the seller.

The soil type used is highly important in the cultivation of Native American herbs, or any herb for that matter. If the herbs have been grown in contaminated soil or in a wrong soil type, their medicinal properties would have been lost or reduced to a bare minimum. You'd only be consuming junk if you take them and this can even be detrimental to your health too.

You can then go ahead to find out the cultivation method and practices used in growing their herbs. Is the herb soil-based or hydroponically grown? What fertilizers did they use? How did they manage pests (the chemicals used)? Ask them the following questions and confirm they're true, whether you're buying from a local or modern producer.

You also want to look at how the herbs were processed after harvest. This part should be seriously looked into because, for most herbs, this is where the contamination starts. Herbs that have had to pass through high temperatures, during processing, would have lost most of their medicinal properties. You'll be able to know this with the color of the leaves. If the plants are relatively darker than what they should be originally, they have lost their quality.

Storage is also important as well. How have they been storing their plants since they harvested them? This would determine if you're going to buy them or not.

So, whenever you're purchasing from a local producer, confirm from them the soil type they use in growing their plants before making a payment. You can also ask them to test the herbs so you can be sure they're completely free of contamination.

## Cultivation

You can also consider growing your own herbs. There are a number of good growing methods you can use and you'll be able to grow your own plants and save some money as well.

Whatever method you chose, whether hydroponic, indoor, outdoor, soil-based, etc. Make sure your herbs are getting an adequate supply of the following things;

- Adequate lighting;
- Adequate water;
- If you're growing them indoors and in soil, you might want to consider using compost to boost the quality of the soil every now and then;

You'd also want to keep your herbs away from rodents and harmful pests that would damage them over time.

Below are some valuable tips to help you with home cultivation and harvesting of herbs:

- Gather all the necessary information you'll need about the plants before starting to cultivate them. If you must cater for a plant, you must be able to understand everything about it. What its needs are, as well as some other information that will ensure you have a bountiful yield at the end of the day.

  You'd also need information about the best practices to follow when growing any plant. The type of fertilizers to use, those to avoid and many other relevant information.

- Growing your own native herbs yourself doesn't only give you the opportunity to save money on a purchase, it also allows you to, in a way, beautify your home as well. Many Native American herbs, if grown indoors, can add bright colors to your living space. Best herbs for this are perennial plants like echinacea.

- Tend to your plants regularly. Don't leave them to die after planting them. Plants like pets also need to be cared for you need to water them, ensure they're getting the sufficient amount of lighting they need, etc.

## Wild-crafting

Some herbs are considered weeds, which means they can be collected directly from their environment from bushes, trees, or other places they naturally occur. These wild crafted herbs work just as fine as the organically grown ones. They are, in fact, the best because they grow naturally and have not been exposed to such things as soil pollution or high temperature that could damage most of the beneficial contents of the herbs. For example, dandelion offers more benefits when wild crafted, their roots, leaves and flowers possess more medicinal benefits when you weed them rather than buy or even plant them.

However, some of these herbs are known to be endangered. So, it is advised that you grow them instead of taking a hike into the wild to wild craft them. If you must go wild crafting at all, there are a few guidelines you must religiously follow. Below are some important ones to note:

- Follow the abundance. Only harvest from places the kind of herb you're looking for can be found in bulk.
- Confirm the herb you're about to wild craft is not listed among threatened species of herbs. This way, you'd be contributing to society and life in general.
- Be reasonable in your wild crafting, don't over-harvest any herb. It doesn't matter if the plants are not endangered, only

collect herbs in small quantities. The quantity you'd need per time would be the most reasonable size of herbs to collect when wild crafting.

- Do not fully harvest mature and/or seed-producing plants. Go for the smaller plants to harvest;

## Storing Herbs

Herbs are delicate "creatures", so to say. They tend to lose their medicinal properties bit by bit, and more quickly when left to sit without drying or processing them. The best way to ensure all the properties of the herbs you should get remaining intact until the time you'll need them, is to store them by drying.

Herbs retain their strength when they're stored in a cool, dark and airtight place. You will even discover that most producers and sellers store their herbs in large containers to keep them safe from oxygen (which can cause them to shrink and lose their power), dust and other external elements that can cause them to lose their properties over time and, eventually, die.

Keep the surrounding temperature on an average, too. Herbs should not be exposed to temperatures over 100°F, or their constituents will reduce gradually until they eventually disappear. Do not expose them to light as it damages the medicinal properties they carry. Best to store them in plastic bags, dark bottles and jars, or glass containers.

A better way to store your herbs, if you have leftover herbs (which you mustn't bin), is to shake them, separate the leaves from the stems, and spread them on a clean, shaded surface. This allows your herbs to get the needed breathing space and also for you to discover and remove every lurking plant pest on the plants.

If you're going to dry your herbs, it's best that you keep the drying period short. The longer the drying period, the quicker the plants lose their power. You can keep the drying frame between 5–7 days for the best results. Make sure they are fully dry to break. This is because the plants, in this mode, can store in their properties and constituents until the time you'd need to make your remedies.

For tree barks, you're expected to carry out a simple process referred to as "tossing." This process involves scraping the outer bark off to remove every polluted part, as well as the pests that have settled discreetly on it.

Roots may require that you wash them to remove every soil particle on them. Once they're clean, you can then store them in large airtight containers.

# Conclusion

Whichever way you decide to source and store your herbs, just make sure you're doing it the right way, particularly for the plant type you're sourcing or storing. There are a lot of herbs, and not all of them would "like to be sourced or stored" in the same way as others. So, it's always great to know your plants before going ahead to source or store them. Some plants are best used immediately after they've been sourced, while other would still do great when they've been stored.

You also have to ensure your plants are completely dry before moving them into storage. Lay them out on a clean, levelled surface they can get ventilation, keep them there until they dry before moving them into your jar. Once in the jar, make sure the place you're storing them next is dry, with a temperature level that doesn't exceed 100°F. Like I mentioned earlier, plants' exposure to heat causes them to deteriorate faster. So, when you're storing them, you want to avoid high temperatures as much as possible to be able to harness the healing power they possess.

# CHAPTER THREE: HERBAL PREPARATIONS

S ignificant in herbal medicine is the way we process the herbs into consumables our bodies can easily absorb. And, all thanks to modern technology, there are easier and quicker ways to extract, purify, and distil herbs to make them "standard" medicines that a larger percentage of the world now consumes today.

However, you really don't have to worry about these "modernised" methods to make the herbal remedies we will soon be looking into later in this book. There are a number of simple preparation methods you can use to get the best results with these herbal remedies. We are taking you back in time to some of the effective preparation methods the ancient Native American used and also add some others that were developed over time.

In essence, this is the chapter you will learn the different preparation methods and processes, the tools you'd likely need to make any remedy, common ingredients added to the herbs, and how to apply some remedies properly

# Methods and Processes

- **Brew/Infusion**; This is usually used in making herbal teas. It's just as simple as pouring boiled water on the herbs, (either fresh or dried). This water *infuses* the leaves and extracts the components you'd need from the herbs. To make this for yourself, pour 2 tsps of fresh or dried herbs into a cup, boil some water and add the water into the cup. Leave to *brew* some time before taking.

- **Decoction**: This method involves boiling some herbs in water over medium heat to dissolve and extract the healing properties contained in the plants. Decoction is always used on hard plants like seeds, tree barks, stems and roots.

  To prepare a remedy for yourself using this process, put sufficient herbs in a small-sized saucepan, add cool water on the herbs, boil the water over medium heat, let it simmer for not more than 40 minutes. Turn off the heat and let it cool for a while before consuming.

- **Percolation**: This is a process similar to that we follow when we make coffees. It involves grinding your herbs (dried), dropping some water or alcohol on the ground herb to moisturize it and then leaving it to sit for a while (about 12—24 mins). After a while, drip water through the ground herb mixture using a valve, a percolation cone or a filtered container. Let the liquid drip till you have a sufficient quantity and consume.

- **Tincture**: like percolation, this process involves soaking, but primarily in alcohol, glycerin, cider or vinegar. What this does is to extract the active herbal constituents from the plant parts into the liquid they're soaked in. Tinctures usually contain more than one herb to ensure a heavy concentration of the herbs' active ingredients. To make this, you'd have to soak the herbs in any of the chemicals or liquids for up to 2 weeks before separating the liquid and consuming.

- **Dual (Double) Extraction**: As with tinctures, you'd also need alcohol in dual extraction too.

  Double extraction is a quite simple process even though the name sounds technical. All you need to do is:
  - Fill a container with your herbs;
  - Add some alcohol in the container until it slightly covers the herbs;
  - Let this mixture sit for about 2 weeks or more;
  - During the waiting period, make sure you shake once or twice every day to combine the active ingredients;
  - After speaking for that duration, strain off the alcohol content and set aside. This is your first extraction.
  - For your next extraction process, simmer the herbs in water for about 30 mins or more. Drain this water into your first extraction and let it sit until cool before taking.

- **Fomentation**: to prepare your herbs with this process, you must have decoted or infused your herbs. Once you have a sufficient amount of the preparation ready, you can then dip a cotton into the alcohol content and dab around the injury area. (**Caution**: This application is likely to irritate your skin and make it go red, so apply minimally).

- **Poultice**: grind your dried herbs into powder, saturate the ground herbs and over the area on your body you'd like to use it.

- **Powder**: all you have to do to make your herbs into fine powder is to grind them dry, without adding any liquid.

- **Oils, creams, lotion, and salves**: you can make this with fresh or dried herbs. You first cook the herbs in oil for some time to extract the oil content. Add beeswax to thicken oil and apply or use accordingly. You can make as much as you'd like and apply on your face or other area you'd like to heal on your body.

# Tools Needed

There are some important tools you'll need to make your herbs too. Without most of these tools, it'd be impossible or extremely difficult and time consuming for you to make the best herbal remedies you can use. You don't need too many though, all you need are the following tools which you might already have in your kitchen.

- Pots
- Saucepan
- Kettle
- Mason jars
- Wire mesh strainers
- Cheesecloth
- Measuring cups and spoons

- Bottles
- Labels
- Valve
- Blender
- Mortar & Pestle
- Cotton cloth
- Knife
- Scissors

The following tools may make things easier for you but are not totally necessary

- French press
- Thermos
- Press pot
- Herb grinder/coffee grinder

# Common Ingredients Used in Herbal Preparations

For most herbal preparations, you do not need more than the herbs and some water. But for some others, you need more ingredients to get the best out of the herbal plants you're using and also to make some herbal remedies easier to apply. These ingredients include:

- **Alcohol**: Alcohol is a powerful material used in forcing out the hidden properties in plants. This is why it's commonly used on herbs to extract their herbal constituents.

- **Apple cider vinegar**: This variant is preferable than the common distilled white vinegar if you're going to be infusing your herbs and/or applying them directly on your body.

- **Honey**: aside from its medicinal benefits, unprocessed honey can serve as wonderful preservatives in your herbs.

- **Oils**: olive oil, almond or grapeseed, cocoa butter, shea butter, lanolin, tallow, and lard are great oil variants you can use in preparing your herbal remedies.

- **Beeswax**: you'll need beeswax for oils, creams, lotion, and salves.

- **Witch hazel extract**: this ingredient is also a great addition to some of your herbal remedies, especially those for topical application.

- **Rose water**: rose water is usually used for skincare and is commonly used to make herbal remedies meant for skin healing and repair.

- **Sea salt and Epsom salts:** salts also, to a great extent, enhance the healing properties of herbs.

- **Gelatin capsules**: with these, you can make your own Native American herbal drugs into capsules. Grind your herbs into powder, and fill the capsules with the powdered herbs before swallowing.

## Methods of Application

We already discussed some of the most common methods you can use to process your herbs. In this section, we will briefly discussing some application methods for Native American herbs.

- **Facial Masks**: Using some Native American herbs like chamomile flow, elder ginger root, ginkgo biloba, ginseng and licorice, you can also make your own facial masks. These herbs are known for their power to remove any excess oil on your face, soften your skin, reduce pores, and completely heal your skin. You can even combine two or more of these herbs to liven up your skin color, smoothen it, and remove all blemishes.

- **Hair And Skin Care:** You can also use Native American herbs to make oils, creams and lotions to apply on your body. Milk thistle seed, rose, and sage leaf are great anti-aging herbs you can use on your skin to promote skin smoothness, softness, and refresh your skin as well.

For your hair, you can use them in making homemade shampoos for cleansing your scalp and ejecting every hair shaft residue that might have been left by modern hair care products you've used. Instead of the chemical-based hair care products that can damage your hair over time, you can use these herbs. Native herbs also offer quicker remedies to dandruff, lice and other related hair conditions too.

- **Poultices, Oils, Salves And Balms**: herbs can also be made into her herbal poultices (by grinding and slightly oiling them) and applied around my open wounds, painful joints, and other affected areas using a cotton cloth or some other "gentle" material.

Herbal oils, when compared to the processed ones, are a lot more affordable. This is why it'd be really great if you have your herbs soaked in olive oil or some other oil type we mentioned in the previous section to extract the medicinal contents of herbs and have them mixed with the oils to be applied as ointments and salves.

- **Baths:** instead of applying the herbs on your skins as creams and lotions, you can as well make them into bathing soaps.

Native American herbs like calendula flower, coneflower, and echinacea work great in treating burns, rejuvenating the skin.

- **Teas:** this is where the process we talked about earlier, infusion, comes in. Herbs can be "infused with their medicinal properties" and consumed as warm or cold delicious teas. This method of use is highly recommended for delicate plants that might lose their contents easily with heat or the addition of alcohol.

- **Tinctures**: Herbs can also be concentrated in alcohol, glycerin, or vinegar and consumed directly either warm or mixed with juice. They might taste a bit bitter but would be easily absorbed into your body.

- **Scents & Fragrances**: Some native herbs can also be used as body fragrances because of the smell great they possess. They can even be used to treat your environment. Just as I'd say, "the way you smell is the way people would see and address you." If you and your environment don't smell great, it'd be difficult for people to come close to you, both physically or emotionally.

Fragrances, however, are usually highly expensive and this can be discouraging most of the time. What we don't know is there are some nature-given herbs we can use to make ourselves smell better. Sage, sweetgrass and pow pow are three of these commonest herbs. They're perfect for every occasion and are usually adopted by perfumers as well.

# Caution

People often assume since herbal medicines are "natural" (which of course they are) they do not have any side effects whatsoever and can be used excessively. But, NO, herbal remedies cannot be used excessively. Herbal medicines, like modern drugs, also have their own side effects which usually don't surface until you overdose on the herbs, make or use them wrongly. This is why I'd strongly advise you consult with a herbalist or any health professional you know to enquire about the right dosages to use as well as the potential side effects that might appear when you take them wrongly.

For example, an overdose of raw elderberries can cause some serious reactions. Another herb is St. John's wort which, according to research, can react wrongly with antidepressants.

Research has also confirmed that some herbs are really dangerous for pregnant and nursing mothers and should be avoided for their safety.

So, in whatever herbs you use, be sure you're using rightly before going ahead to use the remedy. Below are some safety tips to help you make the best use of the herbal remedies you'll be learning how to create later in this book, *Native American Herbalism*.

- There are some Native American herbs pregnant people and nursing mothers have been advised not to consume. Herbs like the American Ginseng and rosemary have been said to affect hormone levels in some and cause uterus contractions in others.

- Avoid giving kids under age 2, who have yet to fully develop their liver, alcohol-based herbs, to avoid serious health complications in the kids.

- Some herbs must not be combined with other drugs. So, if you're taking other medications, consult with a herbalist to find out if you can combine your medications with the herbs. Herbs like Echinacea Garlic, Ginkgo biloba, Licorice root, and St. John's wort must not be used with heart disease medications. So, it is important that you see a medical practitioner to know what is appropriate before taking any herbal remedy.

- Herbs like St. John's wort, etc., should be avoided for people who have medical conditions like asthma and epilepsy. The herbs can react negatively with drugs and also increase the risk of seizures in epileptic patients.

- Always buy your herbs from regulated stores to ensure they are not contaminated or that they've not lost their healing properties with time. Wherever you buy from, ensure the packages are properly labeled and safety information attached. Watch out for the packages too. Always go for herbs in dark packages or those stored in jars and glass. Avoid herbal manufacturers that don't provide adequate proof or information about the quality of their product. If you're in the US, always go for herbs that have been approved by regulatory agencies like NSF International and/or U.S. Pharmacopeia.

# Summary

In this chapter, we've discussed the herbal methods of preparation, application as well as the safety tips for taking these herbs. Next on the line of action is to discuss these herbs themselves. What are the Native American herbs we have been talking so much about and what are they usually used in treating? Let's find out together in the next chapter.

# CHAPTER FOUR: MEDICINAL PLANTS OF NATIVE AMERICA

From the title of this chapter, you might have guessed we'd be briefly going over some of the medicinal plants of Native America. There are more than a 100 Native American herbs and we can't fully exhaust them all in this chapter. However, we'll try as much as possible to go over some of the most common ones you can easily find around you.

Many of us don't know this; but there are so many alternative herbal medications to the modern medicine we have today and we can use them in curing virtually all types of diseases. Many would like to believe herbal medicine is, in their words, "unfounded" (i.e. not backed up by research), but, contrary to this belief, we have a continuously growing body of research on herbs and their uses, and there's scientific evidence that herbs possess powerful healing attributes. Modern medicine didn't even start until the 18th century, after the Industrial Revolution. Prior to this time, people all relied on herbal medicine and if the ancient Native Americans (and all other ancient people) could survive on herbs, why wouldn't we also? A question to reflect on...

**Agave (agave Americana):** the juice from the agave plant is what is used in making the agave nectar, a sweetener used in place of honey or sugar in foods and drinks. This plant helps with body metabolism, strengthens the heart and treats depression. Agave is also one of the safest herbs for pregnant women. It helps to improve their health and that of their baby, too.

**Alder (alnus):** alder barks are infused or decocted and used in treating bleeding gums, throat & mouth inflammation, and also throat pain. It's also used in making lotions and poultices because they work against all sorts of skin conditions like infected wounds, burns, eczema, and hemorrhoids. Native American folktales confirm alder to be a powerful aphrodisiac too.

**Aloe (aloe barbadensis):** like a number of other Native American herbs, Aloe can be used for a range of medical conditions. It heals burns, improves digestive systems, promote good oral health, clears acne and smooths the skin, and relieves anal fissures. Want increased sexual energy? The regular consumption of Aloe can enhance your libido and increase your sexual performance.

**Amaranth (amaranthus sp.):** Amaranth is one of the most common and most nutritious herbal grains Native Americans were generous enough to hand over to us. This plant is high in fiber, antioxidants and other micronutrients. It's commonly used to facilitate weight loss, treat inflammation, and reduce cholesterol levels.

**Angelica (angelica atropurpurea):** this plant is particularly common in Arkansas, USA and is usually mixed, by the natives, with tobacco for smoking. Angelica would be the perfect herb to use if you have menopause symptoms, a cold, arthritis, etc. It can also be used in treating respiratory problems and cancer as well.

**Arrow wood (viburnum dentatum):** is great for treating cramps and inducing vomiting.

**Wild Anise (Myrrhis odorata):** every part of the wonderful plants is useful. The plant works against digestive and intestinal problems, runny nose, and cough. It also works as a diuretic and stimulates appetite.

**Balsam Fir (abies balsamea):** this is commonly used as remedies to external wounds, bites and sores. It can also be taken to heal sore throats, treat colds and other related illnesses.

**Barberry (berberis genus):** Barberry is a great herb to use to aid kidney stone removal and treat kidney pain.

**Bearberry (Arctostaphylos uva-ursi):** among all the Native American plants, Bearberry is quite special. It's what you can refer to as "small but mighty." Bearberry, just as its name suggests, is a low-growing plant with strong therapeutic powers. Extracts from this herb can be used to treat urinary inflammation, bacteria in the urinary tract, and menstrual problems. It works well as an astringent too.

**Black Gum Bark (nyssa sylvatica):** Offers instant relief to chest pains and other pain related conditions as well.

**Bloodroot (sanguinaria canadensis):** juice is usually extracted from this plant to treat fever, respiratory problems, sore throats, rheumatism, asthma, lung diseases, laryngitis, bronchitis, swellings, skin growths, etc.

**Candle Bush (cassia alata):** this plant is used in treating fungal infections. So, you can apply this on your body and face. They can also be used to treat asthma, fever, stomach upset, syphilis, gonorrhoea and even snake bites.

**Cascara Sagrada (Buckthorn):** botanically known as *rhamnus purshiana*, has been used for thousands of years as a natural laxative.

**Catnip (napeta cataria):** Native American used this plant to treat conditions like hives, cold, cough, fever, arthritis, and viruses. But nowadays, people use it for so much more. Catnip is infused and taken to treat illnesses such as anxiety, nervousness and accompanying conditions like insomnia and digestive problems. People also use this plant as treatment for gastrointestinal upsets, and other related conditions like gassing, indigestion, and cramping. Like most of the plants of Native America, Catnip is also a diuretic and it can be used to enhance urination, reduce water retention and treat a lot of other similar conditions.

**Cattail (typha latifolia):** if you're very familiar with herbal medicine, generally, then you must have heard the name "cattail" before. It is one of the most popular Native American plants that's used in foods and also in making herbal medicines. Cattail works well in aiding digestion, refreshing the body, healing wounds and toothaches, and also preventing cancer. They are also used as skincare because of the antiseptic properties they provide.

**Devil's claw (harpagophytum):** this name may seem dangerous but Devil's Claw is far from anything "dangerous." In fact, it's one of the most versatile Native American herbs you'll find. Devil's claw has been used over time by Native Americans to treat various conditions, ranging from fever, to indigestion, to arthritis, to even some skin conditions. The tea can also be used in treating diabetes, gout, back pain, sores headache and reducing swelling joint diseases.

**Dogwood (cornus florida):** the bark of this tree is used in treating different types of conditions, among them is fever, cold, and colic.

**Elderberry (sambucus canadensis):** Can be used in treating all types of medical conditions like headache, indigestion cold, etc.

**Geranium (geranium sp.):** Known for its astringent effects and popularly used in treating fungi diseases like thrush that mostly affects kids.

**Ginseng (panax ginseng):** Another powerful plant gifted to us by the Native Americans, it's used in treating cramps, headaches, asthma, emphysema, menstrual problems and even stroke.

**Golden Alexander (Zizia Aurea):** the leaves, stem and root of this plant can be used as remedies to inflammation, sores, menstrual disorders, psoriasis, vitiligo, etc.

**Heal-all (Prunella Vulgaris):** was regarded, by the ancients, as "the holy herb" the good God sent to us humans to all our diseases. Contrary to the name it carries, Heal-all doesn't exactly heal all diseases, but it can be used to treat several types of conditions such as fever, tiredness, diarrhea, internal bleeding, sore throat & mouth, and liver and heart weaknesses. It has been found to be a highly useful agent in research for serious conditions like cancer, AIDS, diabetes, herpes, etc.

**Honeysuckle (lonicera)**: Has multiple healing properties. It can be used in treating hepatitis, asthma, arthritis, mumps, rheumatoid, pneumonia, and infections on the upper respiratory tract.

**Wild American Licorice (glycyrrhiza lepidota):** The licorice root is famous for its refreshing effects and has long been used in foods, beverages and candies. Herbalists use this toot to treat such illnesses as fatigue, stomach upset, food poisoning, and bronchitis.

**Pipsissewa (chimaphila umbellata):** this plant commonly known to be a "blood purifier," can be used in treating gonorrhoea, blisters, arthritis (and other related conditions), sore eyes, backache, sore muscles, etc.

**Evening Primrose:** A.K.A EPO is extracted from plant seeds. It's used traditionally to cure sore throat, digestive disorders, bruises and hemorrhoids but its use has grown over the years to the treatment of skin problems like acne, and eczema. EPO helps to improve the skin, improve the heart, alleviate depression, reduce breast pain, reduce HBP, minimize hot flashes, ease bone & nerve pain, etc.

**Red Clover (Trifolium pratense):** This plant has been used over the years by to treat respiratory ailments and inflammation. Red clover has also been confirmed to prevent heart conditions and it does this with the reduction of cholesterol and the improvement of blood circulation.

**Saw Palmetto (serenoa repens):** Commonly used for food, but has long been adopted as herbal medicines for treating indigestion, inflammation and abdominal pain. It also helps to stimulate appetite.

**Greek Valerian (polemonium reptans):** the aboriginals used this to induce vomiting, excessive sweating, eczema and epidermis inflammation.

**White Hellebore (veratrum viride):** used mainly in treating external wounds and pain.

**Willow (salix sp.):** Both the bark and leaves of this tree can be used to treat pain and aches.

**Wild Rose (Rosa):** this name might be gentle on the tongue, but I assure you, it possesses strong power to kick out certain diseases from the body. Wild Rose's used by Native Americans to cure common cold and sore throats. Wild rose tea can also be used in treating hypertension, kidney diseases and stimulating the bladder.

**Yarrow (achillea millefolium):** The Native American people used this herb to excess bleeding. This is why it's made into poultices and applied topically around open wounds to help clot blood. Yarrow was also used to heal stomach upset, digestive tract disorders and improve the function of the intestines.

**Yucca (yucca filamentosa):** is one of the plants commonly used in foods by the Native American. It's also used as a treatment for diabetes, Colitis, migraines, headaches, stomach problems, high cholesterol, liver and gallbladder disorders, osteoarthritis, and hypertension.

Some other Native American herbs include:

| | |
|---|---|
| Black Cohosh | Mullein |
| Black Haw | Nettle |
| Blueberry | Oak |
| Boneset | Oregon Grape |
| California Poppy | Pasque Flower |
| Chamomile | Passionflower |
| Corn | Peppermint |
| Cranberry | Pine |
| Dandelion | Plantain |
| Echinacea | Prickly Pear |
| Wild Ginger | Purslane |
| Goldenrod | Red Root |
| Goldenseal | Sage Shrub |
| Gooseberry | Sassafras |
| Gravel Root | Saint John's Wort |
| Hawthorn | Seneca |
| Hops | Snakeroot |
| Horsetail | Slippery Elm |
| Juniper | Usnea |
| Lady's Slipper | Watercress |
| Lemon balm | White Poplar |
| Lobelia | Witch Hazel |
| May apple | Wormwood |
| Maple | Yellow Dock |
| Milkweed | Yew |
| Mint | |

# CHAPTER FIVE: HERBAL REMEDIES & RECIPES

## Abscess

This is what is regarded as the accumulation of pus. It can be very painful and it often leads to fever, swelling of the region affected and redness. It usually occurs on the skin and around tooth gums. The best treatment is to use your herbs as it is highly effective and doesn't present any side effects (if used appropriately) like some modern drugs. However, if things get worse, seek medical help immediately.

### Fresh Yarrow Poultice

| Ingredients |
| --- |
| • 2 tsps of fresh Yarrow leaves |

| Tools Needed |
| --- |
| • Poultice |
| • Clean cotton cloth |
| • Knife |

Instructions

1. Get the chopped yarrow leaves and apply them to the abscess, use a cloth to cover and leave it for 15-20 minutes;
2. Do it twice a day, and let it be for the time frame;
3. Stop only when the abscess has healed.

## Advice

- If you notice any unusual changes on your body or any reaction at all, stop the use immediately. Pregnant women and nursing mothers are also advised to stay away from this herbal medicine.

## Echinacea and Goldenseal Tincture

| Ingredients |
| --- |
| • 10 oz. of dried Echinacea root |
| • 6 oz. of dried goldenseal root |
| • 4 cups of 90% unflavored vodka |

| Tools Needed |
| --- |
| • 2 pint jars |
| • Cheesecloth |
| • Funnel |
| • Dark-coloured glass bottles |

### Instructions

1. Put Echinacea and goldenseal into a well-sterilized pint Jar, add the vodka in until it tops the jar and then, cover the jar with a veil;
2. Get the cheesecloth, use it to cover the mouth of the funnel and pour the mixture through the funnel into an entirely new pint jar;
3. Afterwards, tightly squeeze out the water from the cheesecloth until little to nothing is left in it;
4. When fully prepared, take just 12 drops 3 to 4 times daily for the duration of 10-12 days.

- Diabetic patients should stay away from this herbal remedy. One of its contents, goldenseal reduces blood sugar levels.
- This remedy mustn't be used by pregnant women.

## Acne

This happens when the sebaceous glands get infected, and as a result, shoots out painful bumps—what we all call "pimples." Acne affects all age groups and can appear on any part of the body.

### Witch Hazel Toner

| Ingredients | Tools Needed |
|---|---|
| • <u>3 tbsps</u> of Rosemary oil | • Coloured glass bottle(dark) |
| • 1 cup of witch hazel | • Cotton (cosmetic pad) |

Instructions

1. Put all ingredients into a dark-coloured glass bottle and shake;
2. Prepare a cotton cloth, dip this in the mixture, and apply it on the surface affected every morning and evening until the acne disappears from your skin.

# Sage-Chamomile Gel

| Ingredients |
| --- |
| • 3 tsps of powdered sageleaf |
| • 1 cup of water |
| • 3 tsps of chamomile |
| • ⅛ cup of aloe vera gel |

| Tools Needed |
| --- |
| • Saucepan |
| • Cheesecloth |
| • Glass Jar |
| • Cotton |

## Instructions

1. Put the saucepan on a medium heat, add the sageleaf, chamomile and water. Let it simmer, then get it off the heat when it reduces by half;
2. Let it cool for 3 mins;
3. Prepare a cheesecloth, use it to cover the edge of the funnel, then pour all the mixture to the last drop into a bowl through the funnel;
4. Add the aloe vera gel to the mixture, and mix to blend;
5. Pour into the jar and store in a fridge;
6. Every morning and evening, dip the cotton into the mixture and apply on the affected skin.

## Advice

• Anyone who's allergic to any plant type that falls under the same family as sage leaf and chamomile should avoid using this remedy.

# Allergic Reactions

This is an abnormal effect of some substances that cause the immune system to react badly. These substances are found in many things which may include drinks, foods and even the environment we live in.

## Cattail Tincture

| Ingredients |
| --- |
| • 4 oz. of unflavored 90% vodka |
| • 4 oz. of dried cattail |

| Tools Needed |
| --- |
| • Sterilized pint jar |
| • Cabinet |
| • Cheesecloth |

### Instructions

1. Put the cattail in the sterilized pint Jar and add vodka. Make sure it slightly covers the top of the cattail;
2. Replace the jar cap, make sure it tightly covers the jar, then shake gently to mix;
3. Store for about 8-12 weeks and shake to mix twice daily;
4. Dampen the cheesecloth at the mouth of the funnel, pour the tincture into another sterilized Jar and drain till all the water comes out. Dispose of the herbs and sieve into a clean glass bottle (preferably dark-colored);
5. Take 8 drops everyday until mixture finishes. If it's too strong, add some water or juice to dilute.

### Advice

- If you're allergic to anything that falls under the same plant family as cattail, do not use it.
- It's also not suitable for use by pregnant women and nursing mothers.

# Garlic-Ginkgo Syrup

| Ingredients |
| --- |
| • 3 oz. of fresh or freeze-dried garlic, chopped |
| • 3 oz. of ginkgo Biloba, crushed or chopped |
| • 2½ cups of water |
| • 2 cups of local honey |

| Tools Needed |
| --- |
| • 1 saucepan |
| • Measuring cups (glass) |
| • Sterilized jar |

## Instructions

1. Put the garlic and ginkgo Biloba in a saucepan with some water and boil on low heat. Cover it partially and drain some water out of it;
2. Pour the contents of the saucepan into a glass measuring cup then with cheesecloth on the mouth, drain back into the saucepan and wring till there is no water left.

## Advice

- If you're on antidepressants, you're strongly advised not to use this herbal remedy.
- Children under age 10 should only take ½ to 1 tsp of this remedy 3 times per day.

## Asthma

This is when there is a blockage in the bronchial tubes in the lungs, thereby resulting in breathing shortage and difficulty when anything offensive is inhaled.

### Ginkgo-Thyme Tea

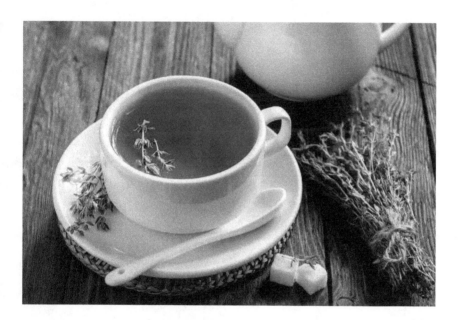

| Ingredients |
|---|
| • 2 cup of boiling water |
| • 1½ tsps of dried Ginkgo Biloba |
| • 2 tsps of dried thyme |

| Tools Needed |
|---|
| • Large mug |

## Instructions

1. Boil water;
2. Pour it into a large mug and add the dried herbs;
3. Allow the tea to steam for 13 minutes;
4. Serve and take your time to enjoy the tea.

## Advice

- Not to be used when on antidepressants.

# Mint-Rosemary Vapor Treatment

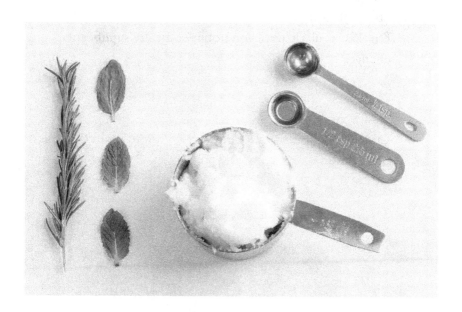

| Ingredients |
| --- |
| • 8 cups of steaming-hot water (not boiling) |
| • 2 cups of crushed fresh mint leaves |
| • 1 cup of finely chopped fresh rosemary leaves |

| Tools Needed |
| --- |
| • 1 large shallow bowl |
| • 1 large towel |

## Instructions

1. Get a big bowl, put the fresh mint and rosemary leaves in it, add the other ingredients including the water, place it on a table and sit facing the mixture;

2. Get a big towel to cover your head and the bowl and inhale the steam coming from the herb;
3. Stop only after the water stops steaming;
4. Do this regularly until you notice some are significant changes.

### Advice

- Epileptic people are strongly advised not to undertake this procedure.

# Athlete's Foot

This is a fungus infection that affects the warm, moist and dark parts of the toe. If not treated as a matter of urgency, it can spread to the toenails and cause discolouration and feet disfigurement later on.

## Fresh Garlic Poultice

| Ingredients |
| --- |
| • 2 garlic pressed cloves |
| • 2 tsps of raw honey |

| Tools Needed |
| --- |
| • 1 small bowl |
| • Cotton-cloth |
| • A pair of socks |

### Instructions

1. Mix garlic and honey in a small bowl. Use cotton to touch the water and apply on affected areas;
2. Afterwards, get yourself the fresh, clean socks pair and rest your feet into them;
3. Let the poultice be on for sometime, for about 30–60 mins;
4. Wash your feet afterwards;
5. You can repeat this twice everyday until your foot heals up.

### Advice

- If you have a skin that reacts easily, you should stay away from this remedy as it could cause skin reactions like rashes, etc.

# Goldenseal Ointment

| Ingredients | Tools Needed |
|---|---|
| <ul><li>2 cups of light olive oil</li><li>4 oz. of diced dried goldenseal root</li><li>2 oz. of beeswax</li></ul> | <ul><li>Medium sized cooker</li><li>Cheesecloth</li><li>Cotton cosmetic pad</li><li>Jar</li></ul> |

## Instructions

1. Set your cooker on low-burning heat, add olive oil and goldenseal and leave for 1 hour;
2. Set aside to cool;
3. Once cool, gently dip the cheesecloth into the mixture, add some infused oil and wrong till it's free from the oil;
4. Dispose of the used herbs and the cheesecloth;
5. Add beeswax to the oil (infused) and let it warm for some time on low heat;
6. After then, when beeswax has melted completely, put it into a very clean jar and allow it to cool;
7. Use cotton to touch the water and apply about 1% of this to the affected area 3 times daily until you're healed.

## Advice

- Not for use by pregnant women and nursing mothers.
- Do not use it if you have HBP.

## Backache

This condition is quite common amongst the elderly. But, most young people also suffer from it, especially those who are stressed or overwork themselves. Besides, inactivity, injury and inflammation can also cause backaches.

## Devil's Claw Tea

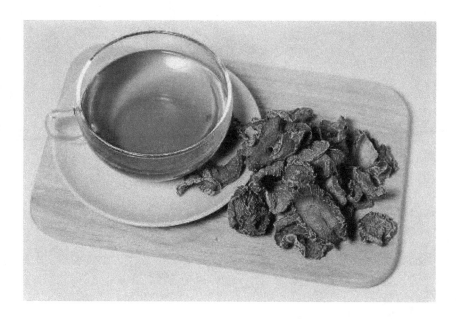

| Ingredients |
| --- |
| • 2 cup boiling water |
| • 3½ tsps of dried Devil's Claw leaves |

| Tools Needed |
| --- |
| • Mug |

## Instructions

1. Boil some water and put the dried herbs into a mug;

2. Add the boiled water into the mug and allow to cool for like 8 mins;
3. Take the tea 2–3 every day until you feel relieved.

## Advice

- Not recommended for pregnant women and nursing mothers.

## Ginger-Mint Salve

| Ingredients |
| --- |
| • 2 cup of light olive oil |
| • 1½ oz. of chopped, dried ginger root |
| • 2 oz. of crushed dried mint leaves |
| • 2 oz. of beeswax |

| Tools Needed |
| --- |
| • Cooker |
| • Cheesecloth |
| • Cotton |

## Instructions

1. Set the cooker on low heat, add olive oil, mint, ginger and leave to cook for 90 mins;
2. Turn off the heat and let it cool for some time;
3. Add some water into the base of the boiler and place on low heat;
4. Put cheesecloth over the top half of the double boiler and pour in the infused oil and leave it on low heat. Ferment some beeswax, add to the mixtures, cook for a while and take off the heat;

5. Pour into a new clean jar and allow it to cool before covering it;
6. Dip the tip of the cheesecloth into the mixture and apply to the affected area (you can also use your finger to apply it);
7. Use this 5-6 times daily, till you're completely healed.

## Advice

- If you are suffering from any gallbladder disease, do NOT use this remedy.

# Bee Sting

This is sustained through bee bite. The area affected often gets swollen and very painful. So, these remedies would reduce their effectiveness.

## Slippery Elm Poultice

| Ingredients |
| --- |
| • 3 tbsps of finely cut fresh slippery elm leaves |

Instructions

1. Apply the chopped slippery elm leaves to the affected area;
2. Leave for 12-15 mins;
3. Use continually, until pain subsides.

# Lavender-Aloe Gel

| Ingredients |
| --- |
| • 3 tsps of dried lavender leaves |
| • 1 cup of water |
| • 2½ tbsps of Aloe Vera gel |

| Tools Needed |
| --- |
| • Saucepan |
| • Sterilized Jar |
| • Cotton Cloth |

## Instructions

1. Pour the lavender into a saucepan, add some water, and boil mixture over medium heat;
2. After some minutes, reduce the heat to low. Make sure the mixture has reduced its water content before you take off the heat. Leave for some time for it to cool;
3. Drape the cheesecloth over the mouth of the funnel and pour the mixture into a jar;
4. Wring the cheesecloth till all water comes off;
5. Add the aloe Vera gel to the mixture and mix to blend;
6. Transfer into a glass jar and cover it;
7. Store in your refrigerator;
8. Apply mixture to the affected area using a cotton cloth.

# Bloating

The major cause of this is overfeeding. Bloating also occurs in some women going through their menstrual periods.

## Angelica-Mint Tea

| Ingredients |
| --- |
| • 2 cups of boiling water |
| • 1½ teaspoon of dried mint leaves |
| • ⅓ teaspoon of ground angelica root |

| Tools Needed |
| --- |
| • A big mug |

Instructions

1. Boil water;
2. Pour it into a big mug, and add the ingredients and let it steam for about 15 mins;
3. Drain the tea into a mug and serve.

# Dandelion Root Tincture

**Makes**: 3 cups

| Ingredients |
| --- |
| • 10 oz. of dandelion root, finely chopped |
| • 4 cups of unflavored 80-proof vodka |

| Tools Needed |
| --- |
| • Pint Jar |
| • Vodka |
| • Cheesecloth |

Instructions

1. Pour the dandelion root into a sterilized pint Jar, add some vodka, ensure it covers the dandelion root slightly, cover the jar tightly and shake to combine;
2. Store it in a cool, dry place and shake 5 times daily for a period of 8-10 weeks;
3. Place a cheesecloth over the mouth of the funnel, then pour the mixture through this cloth into a jar;
4. When done, wring till all the liquid comes off;
5. Take just 2 teaspoons per day for 10 weeks;
6. You can mix with water before drinking if the mixture is too strong for you.

# Bronchitis

This condition is mostly caused by allergies and infections. The area infected gets bloated, becomes really painful and this often leads to constant coughing.

## Rosemary–Licorice Root Vapor Treatment

| Ingredients |
| --- |
| • 8 cups of water |
| • 2 cups of chopped dried licorice root |
| • 1 cup of finely chopped fresh rosemary leaves |

| Tools Needed |
| --- |
| • Saucepan |
| • Bowl |
| • Big size bowl |

### Instructions

1. Prepare a saucepan, pour some water into it, add the dried licorice root and boil over medium heat;
2. Then, let us simmer for 15 mins;
3. After it simmers, pour it into a bowl and add the rosemary leaves;
4. Put the bowl on a small stool, and get a big towel. Cover your head with this towel. Make sure your head faces the bowl directly;
5. Close your eyes during this procedure and inhale the steam from the mixture;
6. Do this again and again until you feel a great improvement.

- Not to be used by people having any of the following; High blood pressure, epilepsy, kidney-related issues, heart diseases and diabetes.

## Goldenseal Syrup

**Makes:** 3 cups

| Ingredients |
| --- |
| • 1 oz. of dried goldenseal root, chopped |
| • 2 oz. of dried hyssop |
| • 2½ cups of water |
| • 2 cups of honey |

| Tools Needed |
| --- |
| • Saucepan |
| • Glass measuring cup |
| • Jar |

### Instructions

1. Place a saucepan on a low heat, add the goldenseal, into water. Leave on the heat until you notice the water has been reduced by half;
2. Pour the content of the saucepan into a glass cup and sieve through a dampened cheesecloth back into the saucepan;
3. Let it boil again for about 2–5 mins, add some honey and stir continuously till fully mixed.

## Advice

- Not to be taken by pregnant women or nursing mothers.
- Not to be used by anyone suffering from epilepsy and high blood pressure.
- Should not be administered to children under the age of 13.

# Bruises

This is a common injury we have on regular days. It could even be a domestic cause like one scratching one's leg over a piece of furniture at home. However, if left unattended to, it could lead to more serious conditions. So, if you find yourself at any point sustaining different bruises use any of the herbal remedies below or contact your doctor.

## Fresh Sage Poultice

| Ingredients |
| --- |
| • 3 tablespoon finely chopped fresh sage leaves |

### Instructions

1. Put the chopped leaves on the affected area, cover with a clean soft cloth, and leave for about 15-20 mins;
2. Do this 3–4 times daily until you're healed.

### Advice

• Not to be used by pregnant women.

# Evening Primrose Salve

| Ingredients | Tools Needed |
|---|---|
| • 2 cups of light olive oil | • Pot |
| • 3 oz. dried arnica flowers | • Cheesecloth |
| • 2 oz of beeswax | • Cotton cosmetic pad |

## Instructions

1. Set the pot on low heat, put the olive oil and arnica in it and let them cook together for 4-5 hours. Afterwards, switch the cooker off to allow the infused mixture to cool off;
2. Put your cheesecloth over the edge of the boiler, pour the infused oil and fold till it gets drained—until there's no more oil left;
3. Put some beeswax into the infused oil and warm gently. When it completely ferments, get it off the heat and pour it into a clean jar for it to cool;
4. When cool, use your finger or a cotton cloth to apply this mixture on the bruised area. Use thrice per day until the bruises are healed.

## Advice

• It can cause skin irritation, so do not apply it on broken skin.

# Burn

Domestic burns can also be cured with herbal remedies.

## Chickweed-Mullein Compress

| Ingredients |
| --- |
| • 3 tbsps of finely chopped chickweed |
| • 1½ tsp of finely chopped fresh mullein leaf |

Instructions

1. Run the plant on the burn and its surroundings and protect it with a soft clean cloth;
2. Let it stay for about 15–20 mins;
3. Do it every 3–4 hrs until the pain subsides.

# Fresh Aloe Vera Gel

| Ingredient |
|---|
| ● Aloe Vera plant |

| Tools Needed |
|---|
| ● Knife |
| ● Cotton |

## Instructions

1. Cut 2–in from the Aloe Vera leaf;
2. Use a sharp knife to cut out the tip, use cotton to take some gel and apply generously on the burn;
3. Do this 3 to 4 times daily.

# Canker Sore

## Goldenseal & Sumac

This helps greatly with surprising pains and helps the healing process faster for internal and external wounds.

| Ingredients |
| --- |
| • 1 tsp of dried goldenseal leaves |
| • 1 tsp of dried sumac leaves |
| • 3 tablespoons of hot water |

| Tools Needed |
| --- |
| • Mortar & Pestle/grinder |

## Instructions

1. Use a grinder or to grind the herbs into soft powder then enclose in a small, thick dark-colored pack;
2. Boil Pack In some water for not more than 5 minutes;
3. Put a very light cloth on the sore, and place the packet over the sore and leave for about 20 mins;
4. Repeat this 2–3 times daily.

# Goldenseal Tincture

| Ingredient |
| --- |
| • 8 oz. of dried goldenseal root, finely chopped |
| • 2 cups of unflavored 80-proof vodka |

| Tools Needed |
| --- |
| • 2 Pint jars |
| • Cotton cloth |

## Instructions

1. Get a sterilized jar, put the goldenseal in it and cover the herb with vodka;
2. Cover the jar and shake gently;
3. Afterwards, store for about 7–9 weeks in a cool dry place, while shaking 2 to 3 times daily;
4. Then, cover the mouth of the second jar with a clean cotton cloth and pour the mixture into a new sterilized jar;
5. Make sure to squeeze the cloth well so all water in it will drain;
6. Pour liquid into a bottle, preferably a dark bottle, and store it in a cool, dry place;
7. To use, get some cotton, dip it into the mixture and apply on the affected areas, about 3–4 drops at once;
8. Do 3–4 times daily until healed.

## Advice

• Do not use this herbal remedy if you are pregnant or breastfeeding.

## Chest Congestion

Or chest tightness occurs when you experience some difficulty breathing well. These remedies would do a lot to clear all those mucus's in the lungs and its pathways.

## Mint & Sage Infusion

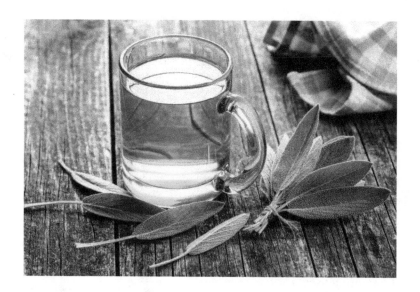

| Ingredients |
| --- |
| • 6 cups of boiling water |
| • 6 tsps of dried mint leaves |
| • 5 tsps of dried sage leaves |

| Tools Needed |
| --- |
| • Teapot |
| • A cup |

## Instructions

1. Put your dried herbs in a teapot, cover with the boiling water and let it simmer for 15 mins;
2. Serve and drink on the spot;
3. You can refrigerate and always heat up again whenever you want to use it again.

## Advice

- Not for asthmatic and epileptic patients, pregnant women, and nursing mothers.

## Angelica-Goldenseal Syrup

| Ingredients |
| --- |
| • 2 oz. of angelica, finely chopped |
| • 2 oz. of dried goldenseal root, finely chopped |
| • 3 cups of water |
| • 1½ cup of honey |

| Tools Needed |
| --- |
| • Saucepan |
| • Glass cup |
| • Jar (sterilized) |

## Instructions

1. Get your saucepan on low heat and add water and the herbs. Let it boil for some minutes, then shift the cover aside;
2. Before you turn off the heat make sure the water in the mixture has reduced by half;
3. Drain the content of the saucepan into a cup and pour, with the cheesecloth, into a new saucepan;

4. Add honey, and put the mixture back on to the heat. Stir continuously without stopping until well mixed;
5. Pour into a sterilized jar and store in your fridge;
6. Take just 2 tablespoons 3 times daily until symptoms stop.

## Advice

- Not to be taken by pregnant women.
- If you're on anticoagulant medications, do not take this herb.
- If you have high blood pressure, avoid this herb as goldenseal shoots up blood pressure.

# Chicken Pox

This is caused by a virus called "varicella-zoster". It is highly contagious and spread uncontrollably if left unchecked. Chicken pox is not curable but it can be managed with herbs until it's successfully suppressed (along with the pain that comes with it).

## Pitcher Plant & Licorice Bath

| Ingredients |
| --- |
| • 6 cups organic unfiltered apple cider vinegar |
| • 1 tsp pitcher plant tincture |
| • 1 tsp licorice root tincture |

| Tools Needed |
| --- |
| • Jar |

### Instructions

1. Get a dry jar, put vinegar and tinctures;
2. Ensure it tightens every well, keep it in a cool dark place till there is need for it;
3. Soak the mixture in a bucket with lukewarm water and have your bath;
4. Do this twice daily.

### Advice

- Anyone with diseases related to blood pressure, kidney disorder, heart diseases and diabetes should refrain from taking this herbal remedy.

# Aloe & Goldenseal Gel

| Ingredients |
| --- |
| • 3 oz. of dried goldenseal root, chopped |
| • 3 cups of water |
| • 3 cups of Aloe Vera gel |

| Tools Needed |
| --- |
| • Saucepan |
| • Cheesecloth |
| • Cotton-cloth |

## Instructions

1. Put the saucepan over medium heat, add water and the goldenseal. Boil for some time and turn the heat down to low. Let it simmer till it has lost about half of the water in it;
2. Remove from the heat and let it cool;
3. Cover the funnel mouth with a clean cheesecloth and drain mixture from the saucepan into a bowl. Squeeze the cheesecloth dry;
4. Add Aloe Vera gel to the mixture and mix to combine;
5. Transfer mixture into a new clean glass jar and cover tightly;
6. Use it for nothing less than 3 times daily using your cotton cloth;
7. Store in a cool dry place when not in use.

## Advice

• Not for use by pregnant women and nursing mothers.

## Cold

The symptoms of this include catarrh, shivering, cough, among others and it's usually caused by certain infections or too much exposure to cold.

## Rosemary Tea

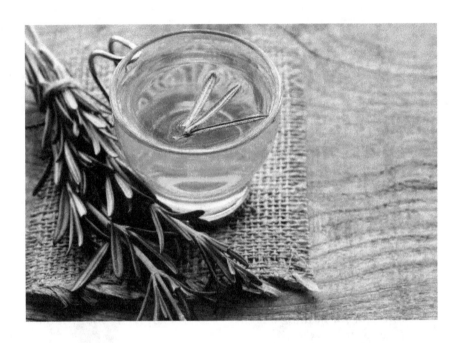

| Ingredients |
| --- |
| • 2 cups of boiling water |
| • 3 tsps of dried rosemary |

| Tools Needed |
| --- |
| • Mug |

Instructions

1. Boil some water, about 1–2 cups;

2. When done, pour into a large mug, add the dried rosemary and cover up the mug;
3. Leave for 15 minutes before drinking the tea;
4. Don't down the tea immediately, just take your time with it.

## Cold Store

This is an infection that affects the mouth and lips, and it is caused by a virus called "herpes."

### Garlic Poultice

| Ingredients |
| --- |
| • 1 garlic clove, cut in half |

**Instructions**

1. Make sure the affected parts are clean;
2. After cutting the garlic into two, use one part to rub the affected area for about 15 mins. Should be done 4–7 times every day.

**Advice**

- If you notice any strange reaction at the earliest stage, halt the usage of this herbal remedy.

# Echinacea - Sage Toner

| Ingredients |
| --- |
| • 1 ounce dried Echinacea root, chopped |
| • 1 ounce dried sage, crumbled |
| • 3 tablespoons of jojoba or light olive oil |
| • 3 tablespoons of Aloe Vera gel |
| • ⅛ cup witch hazel |

| Tools Needed |
| --- |
| • Saucepan |
| • Cheesecloth |
| • Bottle |
| • Cotton |

## Instructions

1. Put all the herbs and oil in your small-sized saucepan, place over low heat and then cook herbs in the oil for about 4–6 hours;
2. Cover a bowl with the cheesecloth, then pour the mixture through it until there is no more oil;
3. Dispose of the cheesecloth and herbs;
4. Then, drain the mixture from the bowl into a dark bottle, add your aloe vera gel and shake to mix;
5. Using a cotton swab, apply around the affected area. Use 3–5 times daily.

## Advice

• If you're allergic to any ragweed plant family, do not take this herb.

## Colic

This condition is common in infants between the ages of 3 weeks to 5 months. Common symptoms include sleeplessness and crying. The herbal remedies below should help reduce the pain. If they don't, visit your doctor again.

### Chamomile Infusion

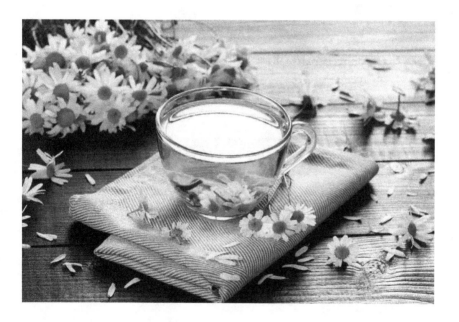

| Ingredients |
| --- |
| • 2 tsps of dried chamomile |
| • 2 cups of boiling water |

| Tools Needed |
| --- |
| • Teapot |
| • Sterilized bottle |

## Instructions

1. Boil two cups of water;
2. Get your teapot and combine the hot water with the chamomile. Let it steep for about 15 minutes after which you should get it off the heat and cool for 5 mins;
3. Once cool, administer only two tablespoons to the baby, twice daily.

## Advice

- If you're on any blood thinners medication, do not use this herb.

# Herbal Gripe Water with Catnip, Ginger and Mint

| Ingredients |
| --- |
| • 2 teaspoons crushed fennel seeds |
| • 1 teaspoon chopped fresh ginger root |
| • 1½ teaspoon crushed dried peppermint leaves |
| • 1 cup boiling water |
| • 1 teaspoon cane sugar |

| Tools Needed |
| --- |
| • Teapot or Mug |
| • Jar |

## Instructions

1. Get a mug, put all the herbs, add water and cover the mug for the herbs to soak for 15 mins;
2. Get the gripe water into the jar add some sugar and fasten the lid and shake till it is mixed;
3. Wait for the water to cool down; then take 2 tablespoons of the mixture and drop gently into the baby's mouth.
4. Do once daily.

## Advice

• Avoid it if your kid has any bleeding disorder.

# Cough

## Cherokee & Mint Tea

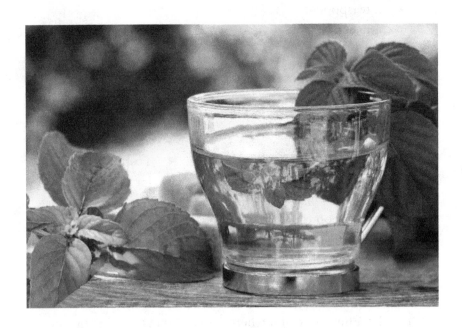

| Ingredients | Tools Needed |
|---|---|
| <ul><li>2 cups of boiling water</li><li>2 tsps fennel seeds</li><li>1½ teaspoon dried hyssop</li></ul> | <ul><li>Boiler</li><li>Mug</li></ul> |

### Instruction

1. Pour the 2 cups of boiled water into a medium-sized mug;
2. Add the herbs and cover the mug for some time;

3. Let it steep for 15 minutes then take the tea slowly while also inhaling the steam;
4. Do this thrice a day.

## Advice

- Not to be used by pregnant women and epileptic patients.

## Licorice-Thyme Cough Syrup

| Ingredients | Tools Needed |
|---|---|
| • 2 oz. of licorice root, chopped<br>• 2 oz. of thyme<br>• 4 cups of water<br>• 2 cups of honey | • Saucepan<br>• Measuring cups (glass)<br>• Sterilized Jar |

## Instructions

1. Set your saucepan over low heat, add the licorice root, some water, thyme and boil with the lids partially open for some minutes;
2. Let it simmer for some time, until it's reduced by half, then pour the mixture into a measuring cup and sieve mixture into another saucepan using a cheesecloth;
3. Add honey to this mixture let cook for some time;
4. Transfer the mixture into a sterilised bottle or jar, put some syrup into the bottle or sterilised jar and store it in a cool place, preferably inside a refrigerator;
5. Take 2 tbsps four times a day until symptoms stops. Dosage for children under the age of 13 should not be more than twice daily.

- Do not take licorice if you're suffering from internal diseases like high blood pressure, kidney-related problems or any heart disease.

# Dandruff

## Echinacea Spray

| Ingredients |
| --- |
| • 2 cups of witch hazel |
| • 2 tbsps of Echinacea tincture |

| Tools Needed |
| --- |
| • Glass bottle |

**Instructions**

1. Put all the ingredients in a dark bottle with a spray top. Shake it well to mix;
2. Apply spritzes to the affected parts 2 to 4 times at once. Use your hand or brush to comb your hair and let it blend well. Leave for 1 -3 hours;
3. Then use shampoo or any other hair soap you have to clean the hair.

**Advice**

- If you, at one point or the other, experience any reaction to Echinacea which is a family of ragweed plants, stop the use of this remedy immediately.

# Rosemary Conditioner

| Ingredients |
| --- |
| • 2 cups of natural, unscented herbal conditioner like Stony brook Botanicals |
| • 55 drops of rosemary essential oil |

| Tools Needed |
| --- |
| • Large bowl |
| • Whisk or Fork |
| • Plastic Bottle |

## Instructions

1. Get a big bowl, put all the ingredients including the essential oil, and use a fork to mix it. Use a funnel to drain it into a Biphenyl-free plastic bottle with a very tight lid;
2. After the application of shampoo, add a small conditioner to the scalp and wait for 3-5 mins before rinsing with cool water.

## Advice

• Do not use it if you're epileptic.

# Diarrhea

## Cherokee Tea

| Ingredients |
| --- |
| • 2 cups of boiling water |
| • 3 tsps dried Cherokee |

| Tools Needed |
| --- |
| • Mug |

### Instructions

1. Boil 2 cups of water, pour it into a big mug and add Cherokee;
2. Leave the tea to steep for about 15 minutes;
3. Drink slowly;
4. Take about 2–3 times daily.

# Catnip-Raspberry Leaf Decoction

| Ingredients |
| --- |
| • 10 cups of water |
| • 4 tbsps of dried catnip |
| • 4 tablespoons of dried raspberry leaf |

| Tools Needed |
| --- |
| • Saucepan |

## Instructions

1. Set your saucepan over medium-high heat, add all the ingredients and water, and boil for 5 mins;
2. Reduce the heat to low, boil for another 10 minutes until water has been reduced by half;
3. Let the concoction to cool before you take it;
4. Pour into a mug and take gently, afterwards put in the refrigerator and let it chill.

## Advice

• Do not use raspberry leaves if it's not well dried, badly processed raspberry leaves have the ability to cause nausea.

# Dry Skin

## Cattail & Aloe Gel

| Ingredients |
| --- |
| • 1 cup water |
| • 1 cup dried cattail |
| • 1 cup aloe vera gel |

| Tools Needed |
| --- |
| • Saucepan |
| • Cheesecloth |

## Instructions

1. Set your saucepan on medium-high heat, add all the ingredients and boil for 5 mins;
2. Take the heat level down to low, and let it simmer until water decreases by half;
3. Turn off the heat and let it cool for a while, put a cheesecloth over the mouth of a funnel and pour the mixture through it into a bowl;
4. Squeeze the cheesecloth dry, into the bowl and add Aloe Vera Gel to the water;
5. Whisk the mixture together to mix then transfer into a BPA bottle and cap tightly;
6. Store in a generator to chill.

# Alder-Lavender Body Butter

## Ingredients

- 1 cup cocoa butter
- 1½ cup coconut oil
- ½ cup jojoba oil
- 2cup Shea butter
- 2 oz. of powdered alder leaves
- 3 oz. of powdered lavender

## Tools Needed

- Cooker
- Cheesecloth
- Hand mixer or blender

## Instructions

1. Get the cooker working, add all ingredients and put the heat the lowest;
2. Allow the herbs to steep for about 4-6 hours then turn the heat and let the mixture cool;
3. Put the cheesecloth over a large bowl and pour the mixture into a bowl through it. Make sure you squeeze out the remaining liquid from the cheesecloth into the bowl;
4. Store the mixture in your refrigerator for it to cool;
5. Get a mixer to mix the body butter with the mixture for about 20 minutes until it's fluffy, then return the bowl into the refrigerator after 25 minutes;
6. Use the tip of your finger to apply it over the affected areas;
7. Stop after you notice positive changes.

# Earache

## Garlic-Cherokee Infused Oil

| Ingredients |
|---|
| • 4 tablespoons of light olive oil |
| • 4 teaspoons of crushed or finely chopped dried or freeze-dried garlic |
| • 4 teaspoons of dried Cherokee flowers |

| Tools Needed |
|---|
| • Boiler |
| • Measuring cup (glass) |
| • Cheesecloth |
| • Small bowl |

## Instructions

1. Boil half cup of water on low heat;
2. Put the garlic, in your measuring cup, add the Cherokee flowers, olive oil, then cook for 4–6 hours;
3. Put the cheesecloth over the mouth of a small bowl and transfer the infused oil into the small bowl with the cheesecloth as a sieve;
4. Squeeze out the oil completely from the sieve then, pour the oil into a new clean bottle with a funnel;
5. let it cool before covering the bottle with its cap;
6. When done, drop 4–5 times into your ear and cover with cotton to protect the drops from seeping out;
7. Leave for 20 minutes and repeat 3–4 times daily.

## Advice

- Garlic may have negative reactions on some bodies, so stop using it if you notice anything unusual.

## Fatigue

This is caused by stress and demanding jobs that drain your whole energy. The herbal remedies below would do the magic by helping you to recover your lost energy so quickly.

### Heal-all Tincture

| Ingredients |
| --- |
| • 12 ounces heal-all |
| • 6 cups 80% unflavored vodka |

| Tools Needed |
| --- |
| • Pint Jar |
| • Cheesecloth |

## Instructions

1. Put the heal-all leave in a sterilized pint jar and add the vodka until it covers the herbs, cover the jar for the herbs to simmer and shake afterwards to mix;
2. Store mixture in a cool, dark place 7-8 weeks;
3. During this period, shake 3 times to properly combine the herbal properties with the liquid contents;
4. Dampen the cheesecloth over the funnel and pour the mixture through it into another sterilized pint jar. Wring and drain the water from the heal-all herb;
5. Then, pour it into a sterilised bottle and mix 12 drops of tincture into a glass of water or juice;
6. Drink this 4–5 times daily until you notice some improvements.

## Advice

- Not to be used by pregnant women and anyone allergic to any ragweed plant.

## Licorice-Rosemary Syrup

| Ingredients |
| --- |
| - 2 oz. of dried licorice root, chopped |
| - 2 oz. of dried rosemary leaves, chopped |
| - 3 cups of water |
| - 1½ cups of honey |

| Tools Needed |
| --- |
| - Saucepan |
| - Measuring cup |
| - Cheesecloth |

## Instructions

1. Get your saucepan ready, place the herbs in and cover with some water. Boil this mixture over low heat, just until you notice the water has reduced by half;
2. Then, turn the mixture from a saucepan into the sterilised bottle using the cheesecloth;
3. wring the cheesecloth dry into the bottle, add some honey to the mix and simmer over low heat, constantly stirring to make sure it doesn't burn;
4. Then, Put some syrup drops into a sterilised bottle and keep it in a refrigerator;
5. Make sure to take just 2 tablespoons four times daily until the symptoms stop.

- If you're diabetic or have high blood pressure, do not take this herbal remedy or any other that contains licorice root.

## Flatulence

It's caused by an increment in dietary fibre and it's often very painful and uncomfortable to live with.

### Mint-Angelica Tea

| Ingredients |
| --- |
| • 2 cups of boiling water |
| • 1½ teaspoons if dried angelica |
| • 1½ teaspoons if dried mint |

| Tools Needed |
| --- |
| • Large mug |

## Instructions

1. Boil some water, add into a mug, then add the dried herbs, cover the mug, let steep for 15 mins;
2. Take tea slowly and inhale the steam as well;
3. Repeat up to 3 times daily until you feel much better.

## Advice

- Not recommended for pregnant women.

# Fresh Ginger & Fennel Decoction

| Ingredients |
|---|
| • 10 cups of water |
| • 1½ tsps of crushed fennel seeds |
| • 1½ tbsps of minced fresh ginger |
| • 3 tbsps of Honey or stevia (optional) |

| Tools Needed |
|---|
| • Saucepan |

## Instructions

1. Set your heat level to high, place your saucepan on it, add water, fennel, and ginger;
2. Let it boil until the water reduces by half before taking off the heat;
3. Allow the mixture to cool;
4. Add some honey, then place in the refrigerator. Drink two cups each evening after dinner;
5. Continue to use remedy until flatulence subsides.

## Advice

• Do not take this herbal juice if you have any gallbladder problems.

# Gingivitis

This occurs as a result of the constant brushing of teeth. This then affects the gum.

## Golden Alexander-Chamomile Mouth Rinse

| Ingredient |
| --- |
| • 1½ oz. of dried calendula |
| • 2 oz. of dried chamomile |
| • 5 cups of water |

| Tools Needed |
| --- |
| • Saucepan |
| • Measuring cup |
| • Cheesecloth |

## Instructions

1. Get a saucepan, add herbs and water. boil over low heat, with the lid partially open, and until the water' reduced by half;
2. Turn the contents of the saucepan into a glass measuring cup, then return the mixture through a dampened piece of cheesecloth back into the saucepan;
3. Wring the cheesecloth until no more water comes out then transfer the mouth rinse to a clean jar or bottle and store in the refrigerator;
4. Take 3 tablespoons per day until this condition stops. But do not swallow this mixture. Children under the age of 13 should take only 1 tbsp of this mixture.

## Advice

• If you've reacted, at any point, to any ragweed plant, in general, completely avoid this mixture.

# Goldenseal-Sage Oil

| Ingredients |
| --- |
| • 2 oz. of dried goldenseal root, chopped |
| • 1 oz. of dried sage, crumbled |
| • 1 cup if coconut oil |

| Tools Needed |
| --- |
| • Saucepan |
| • Cheesecloth |
| • Paper Towel |

## Instructions

1. Combine the herbs and coconut oil in your saucepan, place over low heat setting, cover and slow cook for 4–6 hrs to steep the herbs in the oil;
2. Turn off the heat and allow the infused oil to cool;
3. Drape a piece of cheesecloth over a bowl. Pour in the infused oil, through it and squeeze out the oil from the cheesecloth to the last drop;
4. Transfer the infused coconut oil to a clean, dry jar and allow it to cool completely before replacing the lid;
5. Take 1 teaspoon of this oil and let it melt in your mouth. Make sure it spreads to every part of your mouth around and teeth, but do not swallow;
6. Keep the solution in your mouth for up to 25 minutes at a time;
7. You can take more if you like.

## Advice

- Not for pregnant people and nursing mothers.
- Do not spit oil down the sink since this can clog your plumbing system.

# Indigestion

This is characterized by symptoms such as bloating, belching, stomach ache and discomfort, etc. It often happens when your stomach reacts to something you take. The herbs below should offer you the quick relief you'd need for the symptoms.

## Chamomile - Angelica Tea

| Ingredients |
| --- |
| • 2 cups of boiling water |
| • 2 teaspoons if dried angelica |
| • 1½ teaspoons of dried chamomile |

| Tools Needed |
| --- |
| • Large mug |

### Instructions

1. Boil 2 cups of water;
2. Pour it into a large mug and add the dried herbs into the mug;
3. Let steep for 15 mins. serve and sip gently;
4. Take your time to enjoy the refreshing tastes;
5. Take this 5–6 times daily.

### Advice

- Not to be taken by pregnant women.
- If you're allergic to ragweed, please do not take it.

# Ginger Syrup

| Ingredients |
| --- |
| ● 3 oz. of fresh ginger root, chopped |
| ● 3 cups of water |
| ● 1½ cups of honey |

| Tools Needed |
| --- |
| ● Saucepan |
| ● Measuring cup |
| ● Sterilized Jar |

## Instructions

1. Combine ginger and water in a saucepan then boil over low heat until water is reduced to half;
2. Pour the content into a measuring cup and back to another one through the cheesecloth in order to sieve the liquid. Wringe the cheesecloth until no water is left;
3. Add honey to the mixture and let it boil again on low heat;
4. Then, pour the mixture into a bottle and refrigerate;
5. Whenever you want to use it, shake well and take just 2 tablespoons 4 times a day. Younger children under the age of 13 should take just 2 times per day.

## Advice

- If you're on any blood thinning medication, try as much as possible to avoid this herbal medicine.
- If you have any internal disease like gallbladder disease or bleeding disorder, do not use this remedy.

# Insomnia

This is when one finds it difficult to sleep at night. This can be due to stress or anxiety. Overdose of caffeine can also lead to insomnia.

## Lavender & Hops

| Ingredients |
| --- |
| • 2 cups boiling water |
| • 3½ tsp of chopped dried lavender |
| • 1½ teaspoon crushed dried hops |

| Tools Needed |
| --- |
| • Large mug |

### Instructions

1. Boil 2 cups of water;
2. Pour the boiled water into a large mug and add the dried herbs into, cover the mug and let the herbs steep for a while about 15 minutes;
3. Find a spot to relax and take your tea quietly and slowly;
4. A great time to take this is some minutes before your bedtime.

### Advice

- Do not give to prepubescent children.
- Do not use it during pregnancy.

# Chamomile-Catnip Syrup

| Ingredients |
|---|
| • 2 oz. of dried chamomile |
| • 2½ oz of dried catnip |
| • 3 cups if water |
| • 1½ cups of honey |

| Tools Needed |
|---|
| • Saucepan |
| • Measuring cup |
| • Sterilised Jar |

## Instructions

1. Pour all the ingredients, except the honey into your saucepan, boil over low heat until the liquid content is reduced by half and with the lid slightly open;
2. Then, turn the mixture into your measuring cup and then back into the saucepan using a clean cheesecloth as a sieve;
3. Cook the mixture some more over low heat while stirring occasionally;
4. Once the heat reaches about 110°F, turn the heat off and add the syrup into a sterilized bottle or jar;
5. Store in your fridge for a while before use;
6. Take 1 tbsp ½ an hour before sleep. Children from 10 and below should be administered only 1 tsp 30 mins before their bedtime.

## Advice

- Do not take If you're pregnant.
- Do not take it if you're allergic to the anu plant under the ragweed family.

## Jock Itch

This is an infection that affects the groin, inner thighs and buttocks area. It mostly affects men but is not limited to them. Any areas, which are affected with jock itch can become uncontrollably itchy and painful also painful but the following remedies will provide the needed relief:

### Infused Garlic Oil

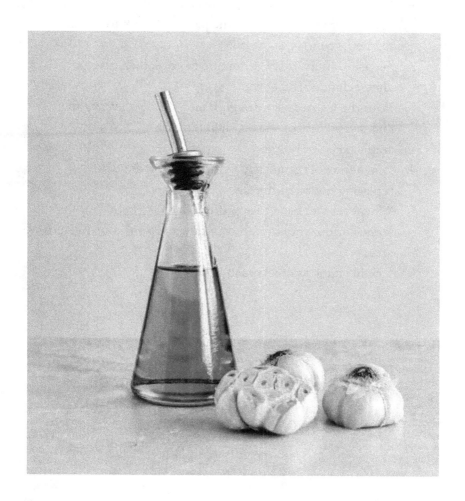

| Ingredients | Tools Needed |
|---|---|
| • 6 oz. of dried garlic, chopped | • Saucepan |
| • 2 cups of light olive oil | • Cheesecloth |
| | • Sterilized Jar |
| | • Cotton |

## Instructions

1. Prepare your saucepan, add the garlic and olive oil into it. Place over low heat, cover the pan, and cook for 6 hours for the herbs to soak in the oil;
2. Set aside afterwards for mixture to cool, then place a cheesecloth over a bowl;
3. Pour the infused oil through it into the bowl, wring the cheesecloth dry of the oil, then transfer oil into a dry, sterilized jar or bottle;
4. Leave to cool completely before capping the bottle or replacing the lid of the jar;
5. Whenever you have to apply, usually 3–4 times daily, dab some cotton wool into the mixture and apply on affected area;
6. Do this until you feel much better.

# Calendula, Chamomile and Goldenseal Spray

| Ingredients |
| --- |
| • 2 tbsps of chopped dried goldenseal root |
| • 2 tablespoons of dried calendula |
| • 2 tablespoons of dried chamomile |
| • 1 cup of fractionated coconut oil |
| • 1½ cups of witch hazel |

| Tools Needed |
| --- |
| • Saucepan |
| • Cheesecloth |
| • Glass bottle |

## Instructions

1. Cook the coconut and herbs for up to 5 hours over low heat, just until the herbs steep in the oil;
2. Turn off the heat and let the mixture cool to room temperature;
3. Cover a bowl with cheesecloth, pour the oil through the cloth into the bowl, rinse the cloth dry and dispose of herbs and the cheesecloth;
4. Pour the witch Hazel and the infused oil into a dark-colored glass bottle with spray top; cover and shake well to mix;
5. Spray this mix on affected areas twice and do this repeatedly 3–4 times daily until you are relieved.

- You can do without goldenseal if you're pregnant or still breastfeeding your baby.

## Keratosis Pilaris

This occurs when the skin produces too much keratin. The skin then becomes dry, rough and bumps begin to appear. It's often detected around the thighs, the back of your arm, armpit and butt line.

### Licorice Root

| Ingredients |
| --- |
| • 1½ cups of baking soda |
| • 1½ cups of crushed dried licorice root |

| Tools Needed |
| --- |
| • Food processor or |
| • Blender |

Instructions

1. Blend baking soda and Licorice in a food processor or blender;
2. Scoop into a bowl and store until ready to use;
3. When about to bathe, take one tablespoon of the mixture and add with your water or body wash and use it to scrub the entire affected areas on your body. Repeat 3–4 times daily until you experience great relief from this condition.

- The baking soda might likely cause dry skin. So, if at the early stage of using this remedy you experience some reactions, stop immediately and consult with a doctor.

## Calendula-Chamomile Body Butter

| Ingredients |
| --- |
| • 3 oz. of dried calendula |
| • 3 oz.if dried chamomile |
| • 1 cup of coconut oil |
| • 1 cup of jojoba oil |
| • ½ cup of cocoa butter |
| • 1 cup of shea butter |

| Tools Needed |
| --- |
| • Saucepan |
| • Cheesecloth |
| • Bowl |
| • Mixer or Blender |

Instructions

1. Pour all ingredients into the saucepan and cook over low heat until herbs are fully infused. This should take a maximum of 5 hours;
2. Once you've done this, prepare a clean bowl and cover with cheesecloth, drain the oil through this cloth into the bowl and wring out the remaining from the cloth before disposing of both the herbs and cloth;
3. Store for a while in your fridge until firm;

4. Whip your butter in an immersion blender. Do this for 10 mins or until butter becomes light and fluffy, then turn butter into your skincare containers;
5. Apply repeatedly to the affected area to get your skin soft and silky.

## Laryngitis

This condition causes the voice box to swell and becomes sore making it impossible to speak clearly or even speak at all. It could be caused by the overuse of the chords, irritation, heavy smoking, etc.

### Slippery Elm Tea

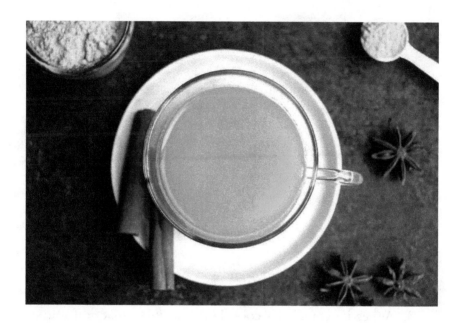

| Ingredients |
| --- |
| • 2 cups boiling water |
| • 2½ tsps of dried slippery elm |

| Tools Needed |
| --- |
| • Large mug |

Instructions

1. Boil a cup of water, pour it into a large mug, add the dried herbs and cover the mug for a while;

2. Let it stay for 15 minutes before serving;
3. Drink tea slowly.

## Ginger Gargle

| Ingredients |
| --- |
| • 2 cups of boiling water |
| • 2 teaspoons minced fresh or dried ginger |
| • 2½ teaspoons honey |

| Tools Needed |
| --- |
| • Large mug |

## Instructions

1. Boil 2 cups of water;
2. Pour it into a large mug and add ginger and honey. Cover the mug and allow the mixture to steep for 15 minutes;
3. When it's completely cooled off, take it like that or if you want it cold, refrigerate;
4. Take three times a day and always keep it cool if not in use.

## Advice

- If you have any bleeding disorder or you're on blood thinning medications, avoid this remedy.

# Menopause

This is a normal change in the function of the female hormone due to maturity. While it is often considered normal, the pain and physical discomfort that comes with it can be quite difficult to handle. But, with the herbs below, dealing with menopause symptoms should be a lot easier for you.

## EPO-Sage Decoction

| Ingredients |
| --- |
| • 3 cups of water |
| • 1½ teaspoons of dried EPO leaves |
| • 1½ teaspoons of sage |

| Tools Needed |
| --- |
| • Saucepan |

Instructions

1. Put all the ingredients in a saucepan and boil over medium heat for 5 mins;
2. Afterwards, reduce the heat and let the water simmer for some minutes until it's reduced by half;
3. Turn off your heat and let the mixture cool for 10–15 minutes before serving and drinking!

# Black Cohosh Tincture

| Ingredients |
| --- |
| • 10 oz. of black cohosh, finely chopped |
| • 2½ cups of unflavored 80-proof vodka |

| Tools Needed |
| --- |
| • Pint Jar |
| • Cheesecloth |

## Instructions

1. Pour the black cohosh into a medium-sized bowl, cover the herb with the vodka. Transfer into a dark-colored glass jar or bottle and store for up to 2 weeks;
2. After this period, take 2 tbsps thrice daily until you feel totally relieved.

## Mental Wellness

There are a lot of things around that can threaten one's peace of mind or mental health. It could be overwhelming career demands, relationship problems, tight schedules and a lot more and this often make one depressed, anxious thus leading to the lack of energy to do anything more:

## St John's Wort Tea

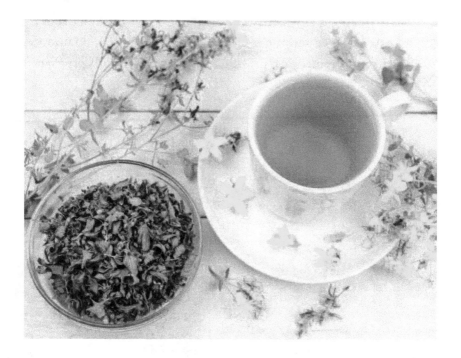

| Ingredients |
|---|
| • 1½ cups of boiling water |
| • 1½ teaspoons of dried St. John's wort |

| Tools Needed |
|---|
| • Large mug |

## Instructions

1. Pour the boiled water into a large mug, add the ingredients and cover the mug for the herbs to steep for 15 mins;
2. Take tea slowly and inhale the steam together as you drink;
3. You can prepare this thrice to four times daily until you feel much better.

## Advice

- If you're on any MAOI (Monoamine oxidase inhibitor) or any selective serotonin reuptake inhibitor (SSRI), do not take this remedy or any other with the St John's Wort Plant.

# Chamomile-EPO Decoction

| Ingredients |
|---|
| • 3 cups of water |
| • 1½ teaspoons of dried chamomile |
| • 1½ teaspoons of dried EPO |

| Tools Needed |
|---|
| • Saucepan |

## Instructions

1. Combine all the ingredients into your saucepan, place over medium heat and let it boil for up to 5 mins. Reduce heat to afterwards and let the mixture to simmer until water is absorbed by half;
2. Let it cool for 10–5 minutes and enjoy your tea.

## Advice

- If you're allergic to ragweed plant, do not take this remedy.
- Not to be used by pregnant women and anyone on blood thinners medications.

# Nausea

This is caused by foodborne pathogens and is usually a precursor to conditions like flu fever and the likes.

## Mint Leaf

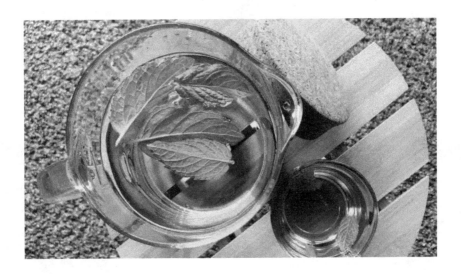

| Ingredients |
| --- |
| • 2½ teaspoons of mint leaves |
| • 2½ cups of water |

| Tools Needed |
| --- |
| • Saucepan |

Instructions

1. Combine the mint leaf and water in a saucepan and boil over medium heat for not more than 15 mins. Turn down the heat to low and let the water simmer until it's reduced by half;

2. Take off the heat and let cool for 10–15 minutes before consuming;
3. Take this remedy 4–5 times every day until you feel better.

## Chamomile-Ginger Tea

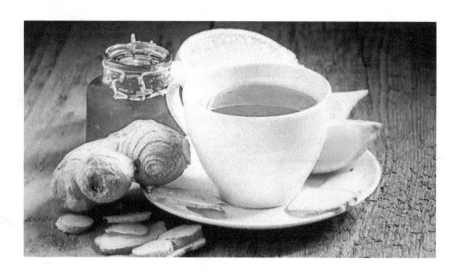

| Ingredients |
| --- |
| • 2 cups of boiling water |
| • 1½ tsps of dried chamomile |
| • 1½ tsps of chopped fresh ginger root |

| Tools Needed |
| --- |
| • Large mug |

Instructions

1. Get a large mug, pour the boiled water and add ginger and Chamomile;

2. Cover the mug for 15 mins tops, just for the tea to steep into the water;
3. Then serve and and enjoy your tea slowly;
4. Also make sure to inhale the steam as it's going to be beneficial to you as well;
5. Do this 4–5 times daily.

## Advice

- Do not use Chamomile if you're allergic to ragweed plants.
- Do not use ginger if you have bleeding disorders or gallbladder problems.
- Also, if you're on any blood thinner medication, avoid using this mixture.

# Oily Skin

This is as a result of excess of sebum, an exocrine secretion that helps in moisturizing the skin.

## Rosemary Toner

| Ingredients |
| --- |
| ● 1½ cups of witch hazel |
| ● 2½ tbsps of rosemary tincture |

| Tools Needed |
| --- |
| ● Glass bottle |
| ● Cotton |

## Instructions

1. Combine all the ingredients into a dark-colored bottle and shake gently to mix well;
2. Using the cotton cosmetic pad, apply mixture on your face 2–3 daily with just ¼ tsps.

## Advice

● Epileptic people are strongly advised not to use this remedy.

# Mint Scrub

## Ingredients

- 2 cups of dried mint leaves, packed
- 1 cup of baking soda

## Tools Needed

- Food processor or blender
- Container

## Instructions

1. Blend the mint leaves and baking soda in a food processor for 10–15 minutes, until the mixture turns fine powder;
2. Transfer the blended powder into a clean contain cover with its lid;
3. Then, clean your face with water, apply about 1½ teaspoons of the powder on your skin and rub the powder in;
4. Do this thrice every day and ensure you clean your face properly after usage.

# Poison Ivy

## Herbal Spray with Calendula, Chamomile and Witch Hazel

| Ingredients |
| --- |
| • 1 cup of witch hazel |
| • 4 tablespoons of calendula oil |
| • 3 tablespoons of chamomile tincture |

| Tools Needed |
| --- |
| • Glass bottle |

### Instructions

1. Add all the ingredients into a dark glass bottle with a spray top, shake well to mix, then apply 2–3 sprays on to the affected area;
2. Do this for 4–5 times daily and ensure the sprayed mixture dries up before you dress up.

### Advice

- Those allergic to ragweed plant family are advised not to use this herbal remedy.

# Licorice Root Powder

| Ingredients |
|---|
| • 8 oz. of dried licorice root |
| • 8 oz. of organic rolled oats |

| Tools Needed |
|---|
| • Food processor |

## Instructions

1. Put all the ingredients into a food processor, then add the chopped Licorice Root into it. Set up your food processor or blender and blend ingredients at a high speed;
2. When ground into fine powder, transfer it into a dry and clean container and cover up;
3. With a brush, apply the power on the affected area and wear a very light cloth over it;
4. Apply 3–4 times daily and continue till there are significant changes.

## Advice

• Do not take if you have any internal disease such as HBP, cardiovascular diseases and kidney-related disorders.

## Premenstrual Syndrome (PMS)

This happens when the monthly menstrual cycle is about to take place. Women often find themselves having mood swings, bloating, headaches, nausea, etc. This makes them uncomfortable both mentally and physically but with the help of the following herbal remedies, they can have relief from the symptoms that come with PMS.

### Dandelion & Ginger Tea

| Ingredients |
| --- |
| • 1½ cups of boiling water |
| • 2 teaspoons of chopped dandelion root |
| • 1½ teaspoons of chopped ginger root |

| Tools Needed |
| --- |
| • Boiler |
| • Large mug |

Instructions

1. Boil just 1½ cups of water;
2. Pour it into a large mug, add the roots and cover for 12 minutes, just for the roots to steep;
3. Take tea slowly and inhale the steam as well. Do this 6 times daily until you feel much better.

Advice

- If you're on medications for gallbladder diseases, kidney-related issues, or blood thinners, do not take ginger.

# Black Cohosh Syrup

| Ingredients | Tools Needed |
|---|---|
| • 3 oz. of black cohosh | • Saucepan |
| • 2½ cups of water | • Measuring cups |
| • 2 cups of honey | • Jar or Bottle (Sterilized). |

## Instructions

1. Put the black cohosh and water together into a saucepan. Boil the water over low heat with the lids slightly open;
2. Leave the water to simmer until the water in the saucepan reduces by half;
3. Then, pour the content of the saucepan into a measuring cup. Cover the measuring cup with a cheesecloth and pour the mixture back into the saucepan through the cheesecloth. Wring the cheesecloth dry and dispose of it;
4. Put the saucepan over low heat and add some honey, then stir gently to mix;
5. Keep in the low heat until the mixture becomes slightly hot;
6. Then pour the syrup into a bottle and store it in a refrigerator;
7. Take 2 spoons daily till the symptoms stop.

# Ringworm

This is a fungal infection that forms circular patches over the affected spot. It's usually accompanied by blister edges and redness. Ringwood is highly contagious and itchy and it can spread to others with physical contact.

## Fresh Garlic Compress

| Ingredients |
|---|
| • 2⅓ cups of steaming-hot water |
| • 2½ garlic clove, cut in half |

| Tools Needed |
|---|
| • Silk cloth |
| • Boiler |

## Instructions

1. Boil 2½ cups of water, soak a soft cloth in it and add garlic clove;
2. Slightly squeeze the cloth and apply it onto the affected areas, press over the affected regions for 15–20 mins, then dispose of the garlic;
3. Repeat this twice daily, with new garlic cloves and cloth.

## Advice

• If you have very sensitive skin, minimize the use of garlic and if there is any effect while you're using this remedy, stop immediately and consult with a health practitioner.

# Goldenseal Balm

| Ingredients |
| --- |
| • 3 ounces of dried goldenseal root |
| • 1 cup of coconut oil |
| • 1 oz. of beeswax |
| • 23 drops of tea tree essential oil (optional) |

| Tools Needed |
| --- |
| • Saucepan |
| • Boiler |
| • Cheesecloth |
| • Tins |

## Instructions

1. Prepare your saucepan and place over low heat, add the goldenseal and coconut oil into cover slightly and cook for 4–6 hours;
2. Turn it off after then and let the mixture cool;
3. Boil some water over medium heat, add to the mix, turn into a bowl, and return into the saucepan through a cheesecloth saucepan, wring the oil in the cloth dry and dispose of it;
4. Add beeswax to the mixture in the pan and let it simmer over low heat for a while until the beeswax melts;
5. Then, put the tea tree essential oil into the boiler and quickly pour the mixture into clean, dry jars or tins and let cool completely before covering;
6. apply over the affected areas 2 to 3 times daily.

## Advice

• Pregnant women and nursing mothers should not use this remedy.

# Sinus Infections

## Yarrow Shot

| Ingredients |
|---|
| • 4 teaspoons of fresh or prepared yarrow or wasabi |
| • 6 tablespoons of water |

| Tools Needed |
|---|
| • Small glass cup |

### Instructions

1. Get a small glass cup or mug, add yarrow leaves and some water;
2. Let it soak for a while, then drink mixture;
3. Repeat 5 times daily.

### Advice

• Stay away from this remedy if you have low thyroid function.

# Mint - Echinacea Tea

| Ingredients |
| --- |
| • 2 cups of boiling water |
| • 2 teaspoons of dried mint leaves |
| • 1½ teaspoons of chopped dried Echinacea root |

| Tools Needed |
| --- |
| • A large mug |

## Instructions

1. Pour the boiled water into a large mug and add the dried herbs;
2. Cover it and let the tea cool for about 7 minutes;
3. Take tea gently while also inhaling the steam;
4. You can take this 5 times daily.

## Advice

- Do not take it if you have any autoimmune disorder.

# Tendinitis

## Ginger Tea

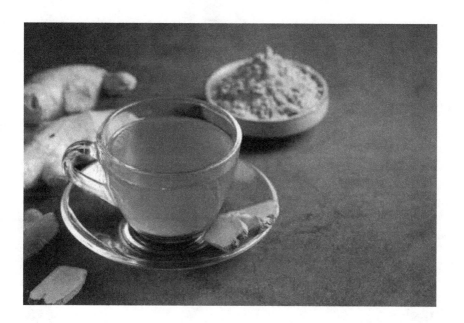

| Ingredients |
| --- |
| • 2 cups of boiling water |
| • 3 tsps of chopped fresh ginger root |

| Tools Needed |
| --- |
| • Large mug |

## Instructions

1. Boil 2 cups of water;
2. Pour it into a mug, add ginger to it and cover it. Let it steam for 15 mins before downing;
3. Take your time with the tea and consume only twice daily.

- Do not take it if you have bleeding disorders or gallbladder diseases.

## Mint Salve

| Ingredients |
| --- |
| • 3 oz of dried mint leaves |
| • 2 cups of light olive oil |
| • 2 oz of beeswax |
| • 25–35 drops of mint derived essential oil. |

| Tools Needed |
| --- |
| • Cooker |
| • Cheesecloth |
| • Boiler |

Instructions

1. Get your cooker working slowly, add the mint leaves and some olive oil into it and cover the cooker, and let it steep for 4-6 hours. Turn it off afterwards and let the mixture cool to room temperature;
2. Pour some water to a simmer at the end of a double boiler and reduce heat to the lowest;
3. Put the cheesecloth over the upper half of the boiler and pour through it, then wring the cheesecloth to the last drop of oil;
4. Add beeswax to the mixture in the boiler, and when the beeswax melts completely, remove the pan from the heat;

5. Turn the contents of the pan into a clean jar and allow it to cool to room temperature before covering the jar with its lid;
6. To apply on affected areas, dip cotton into the mixture and gently touch the region with it;
7. Do this every 3–4 hours.

# Urinary Tract Infection (UTI)

This is a condition that affects the urinary tracts and causes patients great pains during urination.

## Cranberry Tea

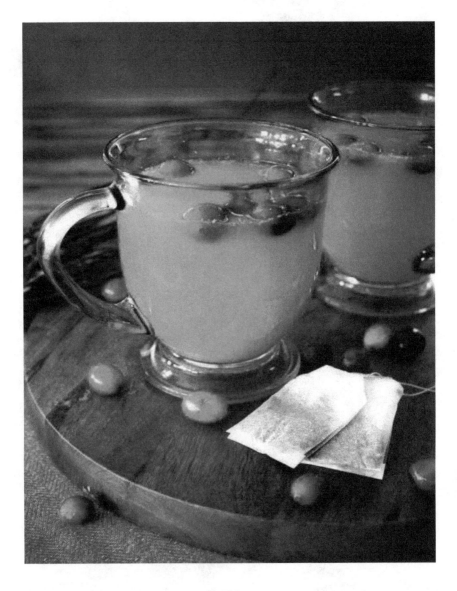

| Ingredients |
| --- |
| • 1 cup grated fresh cranberries |
| • 10 cups boiling water |

| Tools Needed |
| --- |
| • Saucepan |

## Instructions

1. Put all the ingredients into a saucepan and bring to boil. It shouldn't take more than 15 minutes;
2. Turn off the heat and wait for the mixture to cool to room temperature;
3. When cool, pour it into a glass and drink immediately;
4. Take one glass every 3 hours until you notice changes or the pain subsides.

## Advice

• Anyone with low thyroid function should not take this remedy.

# Dandelion Tincture

| Ingredients |
| --- |
| • 10 oz. of dandelion root, finely chopped |
| • 2 cups of unflavored 80-proof vodka |

| Tools Needed |
| --- |
| • Sterilized jar |

## Instructions

1. Prepare a sterilized pint jar, add the dandelion root and cover with vodka;
2. Cover the jar well and shake to mix;
3. Store in a cool, dry place;
4. Cover funnel with cheesecloth, then pour the mixture through it into another pint jar. Make sure to squeeze out the cheesecloth till all the liquid comes out;
5. Transfer water into a glass bottle and always take it from there;
6. Take 1 spoon 4–5 times daily.

# Wrinkles

This is a sign of aging and it isn't unusual. But, the concoction under this section would help to prevent it and if it's already manifesting, would help you manage it well.

## Calendula Toner

| Ingredients |
| --- |
| • 1 cup of witch hazel |
| • 2½ tablespoons of calendula oil |

| Tools Needed |
| --- |
| • Dark-coloured bottle |
| • Cotton |

**Instructions**

1. Put all the ingredients into a dark-coloured glass and shake gently;
2. Using a cotton cosmetic pad, apply 6 drops to your already washed face;
3. Use twice daily.

# Aloe Facial Gel

| Ingredients |
|---|
| • 2 tbsps of Aloe Vera gel |
| • 2 tsps of coconut oil |

## Instructions

1. Clean your face with clean water;
2. Apply some Aloe Vera gel and wait for your skin to absorb then spread coconut oil over it;
3. Dampen a soft cloth in the warm water and spread over your face;
4. Let it rest for 5 minutes, then, use warm water to remove excess coconut oil;
5. Repeat for a minimum of 5 times every week.

# Yeast Infection

## Garlic Suppository

| Ingredients |
| --- |
| • 8 garlic cloves, peeled |
| • 7 tbsps of plain yogurt with live, active cultures |

| Tools Needed |
| --- |
| • Food processor or blender |
| • Container |

### Instructions

1. Combine garlic and yoghurt into a food processor and blend until fine and smooth;
2. Pour it into an airtight, clean container and freeze in your refrigerator until when you're ready to use;
3. Add about $1/7$ of the remedy to an applicator-free tampon, then insert the tampon into your vagina;
4. Leave for 90 mins. Then, remove the tampon after use and dispose of it;
5. Do this thrice daily for a period of 4 days.

### Advice

• If your skin is sensitive, you might want to use this remedy carefully as it can cause serious skin irritation. Be sure you don't react to garlic before you use this herbal medicine.

# Chamomile - Calendula Douche with Echinacea

| Ingredients |
| --- |
| • 6 cups of water |
| • 2 tablespoons of dried chamomile |
| • 2 tablespoons of dried calendula |
| • 2 tablespoons of chopped dried Echinacea root |

| Tools Needed |
| --- |
| • Saucepan |

## Instructions

1. Put water, Chamomile, Calendula and Echinacea in a saucepan and boil the mixture over medium heat;
2. After some time reduce heat and leave it to simmer for a while;
3. When the water reduces by half, remove the saucepan from the heat and leave it somewhere till it cools down;
4. Freeze until needed;
5. Whenever you need to clean your face, with a cotton cloth and apply 2 cups of the mixture in the vagina;
6. Repeat just once after 3 days and you'll start to see some improvements;
7. If the condition persists, consult with your health practitioner.

## Advice

• If you're allergic to the ragweed family plants, do not undertake this procedure.

# Conclusion

We've now come to the end of Native Herbalism.

Now, what next? Taking your time to apply all you've learned in this book. Native American Herbs have long been used to cure many illnesses and conditions. These herbs are still being studied all over the world for their hidden healing properties and will still continue to be used in America and beyond to treat different conditions. So, take your chance with the remedies you've learnt in this book today and begin to live a freer, healthier and more fulfilled life.